Pain Seeking Understanding

Pain Seeking Understanding

Suffering, Medicine, and Faith

Edited by Margaret E. Mohrmann
and Mark J. Hanson

The Pilgrim Press

Cleveland, Ohio

The Pilgrim Press, Cleveland, Ohio 44115
© 1999 by Margaret E. Mohrmann and Mark J. Hanson

Printed in the United States of America on acid-free paper

05   04   03   02   01   99   5   4   3   2   1

Library of Congress Cataloging-in-Publication Data

Pain seeking understanding : suffering, medicine, and faith / edited
by Margaret E. Mohrmann and Mark J. Hanson.
     p.   cm.
   Includes bibliographical references.
   ISBN 0-8298-1354-3 (pbk. : alk. paper)
   1. Theodicy.   2. Suffering—Religious aspects.   3. Medicine and
religion.   4. Medical ethics.   5. Pastoral medicine.   I. Mohrmann,
Margaret E., 1948–   .   II. Hanson, Mark J.
BT160.P17   1999
231′.8—dc21   99-34494
                                                        CIP

Contents

Contributors

Per Anderson is associate professor of religion at Concordia College, Moorhead, Minnesota.

Larry D. Bouchard is associate professor of religious studies at the University of Virginia, Charlottesville.

Ronald Cole-Turner is professor of theology and ethics at Pittsburgh Theological Seminary, Pittsburgh, Pennsylvania.

Julia E. Connelly is professor of medicine and co-director of the Humanities in Medicine Program at the University of Virginia, Charlottesville.

Elliot N. Dorff is a rabbi, a professor of philosophy, and the provost at the University of Judaism, Los Angeles, California.

Wendy Farley is associate professor in the graduate division of religion at Emory University, Atlanta, Georgia.

Mark J. Hanson is associate for ethics and society at the Hastings Center, Garrison, New York.

Deborah E. Healey is associate professor of pediatrics at the University of Virginia, Charlottesville.

Albert H. Keller is associate professor of family medicine (ethics) at the Medical University of South Carolina and pastor of Circular Congregational Church, both in Charleston.

Margaret E. Mohrmann is associate professor of pediatrics and medical education at the University of Virginia, Charlottesville.

James Lindemann Nelson is professor of philosophy at the University of Tennessee, Knoxville.

Daniel P. Sulmasy is director of the Center for Clinical Bioethics at Georgetown University in Washington, D.C.

Introduction: Suffering, Medicine, and Faith

Margaret E. Mohrmann

This is a book about people who suffer and come to medicine for clarification and relief, and about how they may attempt to reconcile the fact of suffering, perceived as the onslaught or consequence of evil in some form, with prior beliefs about divine order and meaning in the cosmos. Thus, broadly speaking, it is a book about theodicy, the theological enterprise of justifying God in the face of evil.[1] The existence of evil challenges definitions of God as both utterly good and omnipotent; the "problem of evil," in theological terms, is the problem of holding simultaneously three apparently contradictory claims: that God is good, that God is all-powerful, and that evil exists. In this introduction, I briefly describe ways that theologians have framed the problem in order to "solve" it; likewise, the authors of some of the chapters that follow present details of various theodicies in order to establish bases or contrasts for their own thinking on the subject.

The book as a whole, however, is not itself intended to be a theodicy. That is, it is not an apologetic work, designed to convince unbelieving readers that evil is no obstacle to belief in a good and powerful God. Nor is this effort directed toward assisting or confirming believers in their particular ways of resolving the dilemma inherent in accepting the real existence of both manifest evil and God as the omnibeneficent Creator. Rather, some of the chapters describe ways in which these seemingly paradoxical beliefs, often unscrutinized and quietly held by many, may clash intolerably when evil comes too close, in the guise of the physical and emotional suffering that attends illness or injury in oneself or in those one loves.

Some of the chapters describe, and prescribe, how different theodicies, different ways of making sense of the paradoxes, may respond to the particular issues embedded in medical suffering. For it is one thing to consider questions of theodicy in the abstract—that is, to reason about God in the face of universal evil, or human suffering in general, or egregious historical manifestations of evil—but it is quite another to work through the problem in the presence of concrete, individual suffering, evil experienced in one's own body or observed in a loved one or a patient, from the perspective of a victim or a survivor or a witness.

The subject, therefore, is how one may comprehend a present reality of evil and its attendant suffering *and* a cosmology or theology that accounts also for one's past and present experiences and perceptions of goodness and meaning.[2] Moreover, this book attempts not only to illuminate that issue of understanding but also to suggest how health care professionals and chaplains—persons attending to those who seek medical relief from their suffering—may be able both to hear patients' consternation about the "problem of evil" and to respond to it in supportive, enlightening, and even healing ways.

Traditional Theodicies

What follows is a brief discussion of various ways in which theologians and religious traditions have resolved, more or less satisfactorily, the logical problem of evil and the nature of God. For the most part, these theodicies are Christian in origin, although Jewish theodicy, except where noted, has not differed remarkably in its premises or outcomes.[3] It is, however, important to note that even explicitly Christian theodicies have many points in common with the ways in which those who consider themselves agnostic or atheist work out their own dilemmas about the way the world works.

Most humans work out or adopt some sort of cosmology, a more or less rudimentary, more or less explicit understanding of how the various aspects of human life and its relation to the universe fit together. Even those who do not call on God, or Jesus, or Allah in times of trial may feel the anguish of having their assumptions—about the benignity of the universe, or its manifest orderliness, or the meaning of their place and significance within human relationships of love and work—broken apart by the advent of personally experienced evil in the form of incomprehensible suffering. The theodicies of organized religion tell us not only something about the beliefs of those particular traditions, but also much about human ways of making sense of universal human experiences of good and evil, order and disorder, hope and pain.

If we begin with the assumption that theodicy is basically concerned with reconciling the apparently contradictory propositions that God (or the cosmos) is both good and powerful, and that evil exists, then it follows that the answers must be ways of "breaking" one or another of the propositions by showing it to be either false or misconceived.[4] Most attempts at solution have focused on the nature of God's power. The "free-will defense"—versions of which prevail historically within Christian theology—proposes that God, in order to create free human beings (who must be free to be in God's image, in accordance with scriptural teachings, and to be creatures whose love, obedience, and worship of God can be meaningful, because freely offered), has to limit God's own power such that humans are free even to choose and/or create evil.[5]

In the Augustinian version of free-will theodicy, arguably the form that permeates most popular understanding of this topic, the "Fall" from created perfection was occasioned by humans' choosing evil, a choice allowed by God for the greater good of human freedom. The Fall is implicated as the progenitor of all subsequent human suffering, and suffering is, therefore, in some sense always deserved, whether directly because it is the result of some person's act of evil, however distant, or indirectly because each human being is so tainted with the universal human choice of evil as to be guilty and deserving of whatever pain evil can inflict. Hope, in this construct, lies only in redemption and eschatological recompense.

A recently revived alternative to the stern Augustinian model of original sin, guilt, and desert is also a variation on the free-will defense. In this approach, based on the writings of Irenaeus, a second-century Christian apologist, God's self-limited power created beings who are not perfect from the start, in contrast to the Augustinian presumption, but who need to grow into moral and intellectual maturity.[6] Suffering is understood both as inevitable—because of human imperfection—and as pedagogical and salutary. It is through suffering that one grows closer to the ideal for which one was created; suffering is part of the perfecting process. This approach, like the Augustinian model, relies on eschatological hope, in this case not as recompense for deserved punishment of the fall from perfection, but as fulfillment of the arduous purgatorial route *toward* perfection.

It is easy to hear in these two free-will approaches echoes of popular notions about suffering. Perhaps the most commonly observed human responses to personally experienced evil are self-examination to discover how the suffering may be deserved and an attempt to see the experience as one by which the sufferer may "grow" in some way. An amalgamated theodicy that includes elements of both desert and growth is often heard from patients regardless of their religious inclinations. This popular theodicy may speak to human urges not to be passive—that is, to claim some degree of accountability for what happens to us— and to turn the evil into good, to postulate a positive effect from negative experience.

Despite the prevalence of this way of thinking, the theodicies attributed to Augustine and Irenaeus have obvious logical and emotional flaws. God's self-limitation of power leaves intact God's omnipotence; God, after all, has chosen not to exercise a power that God in fact possesses. The question that then arises is, How can God be considered utterly good, given God's choice to use or to constrain power in such a way that evil can result? Does human freedom require that there be *so much* evil? Can there be *no* divine limitations on humans' ability to hurt themselves and others? David H. Smith has described the free-will defense as one in which "the characteristic Western preoccupation with freedom is ascribed to the deity."[7] Can we attribute such a "preoccupation with freedom" to God and still be certain of a level of loving protective care from God that can support us in our times of pain?

In response to doubts about God's goodness in the face of the evil God chooses not to prevent, theologians invoke mystery and the eschaton, theorizing that all will be seen to be good when we can grasp the bigger plan. We cannot understand God's goodness from our vantage point, nor see how this pain now can translate into greater good at some point, but we can trust that God's goodness and the goodness of all our experiences will ultimately prove true. This argument, in effect, solves the theodicy riddle by preserving God's goodness and power while breaking the proposition that evil is real. If all will be well eventually, beyond our present capacity to predict or comprehend, then our suffering now cannot matter as much as it seems; from the perspective of eternity, it will not appear to be suffering at all.[8] Whether suffering serves to punish us justly or to teach and perfect us, it is all good (not evil), as part of bringing us successfully to the finish line of salvation without impinging on our freedom.

Besides logical difficulties with these versions of free-will theodicy, there are other significant ways in which they may outrage our senses of self and morality. To begin with, there simply seems to be too much evil for these austere arguments to handle. It is hard for any amount of moral grief over the presumed fall from perfection to accept that *all* human suffering is thereby deserved. One need only consider the agonies of young children with serious chronic disease or crippling injuries to question attributions of desert. To argue that the fault lies with certain adults, who must now suffer by witnessing the child's pain, is once again to make God's goodness untenable. Any humanly intelligible definition of goodness cannot encompass even the deserved punishment of people by the indirect means of torturing those they love.

Just as arguments about deserved suffering falter in the face of certain sufferers and the sheer quantity of human pain, so do theories about suffering's pedagogical value. It is too clear that there are many sufferers who cannot grow from their experience because the event itself is so shattering, physically and/or psychologically, as to destroy any possibility of change or learning. This is not to deny that many people do find suffering to be an occasion of remarkable growth in understanding and in emotional capacity, but this is not always true, nor can it be. Days of ceaseless agony, as from a severe burn, that culminate in a screaming death can scarcely be called a growth experience for the sufferer. Even if those who care for such an afflicted person can somehow mature and become wiser for the experience, their perfecting cannot justify what has happened to the sufferer without irreparably indicting God's goodness. Whose growth could require or, at the least, be assisted by the tortured deaths of millions of Jews or Ukrainians or Cambodians? Arguments from desert or from pedagogy cannot handle the task of justifying God in the face of the magnitude of evil that constantly confronts human awareness.

Since the Holocaust, Jewish theology has had to wrestle anew with the problem of evil, the enormity and inescapable reality of genocide having made earlier, abstract solutions of the sort just described no longer tenable. A more recent "theodicy of protest" has painfully accepted one consequence of previous accounts: God cannot be perfectly good, given the reality of evil. While preserving God's omnipotence, this theodicy calls God to account for the misuse of power in refusing to constrain human evil.[9] Although clearly the comfort of reliance on God's goodness is lost by such reasoning, there may be a beneficial empowering—in contrast to the enervating effects of "consolations" that speak of guilt or growth—of the sufferer, who is allowed to express anger at his or her state by shaking a fist at God and demanding better treatment.

In contrast to contemporary Jewish solutions to the question of theodicy, many present-day Christian theologians respond to the problem of evil—intensified by twentieth-century evidences of genocide, oppression, and pervasive injustice— by emphasizing God's goodness, presence, and participation in human suffering. This move usually includes an unflinching acceptance of—indeed, an insistence upon—the reality and significance of evil and suffering. The classic dilemma is then resolved by breaking the proposition of divine omnipotence. In various ways, God's might is reconceived as partial, although still considerable, with certain aspects of existence remaining outside God's sovereignty, but not by God's choice. Divine power is reinterpreted as power to be present with, to strengthen, hold, and transform sufferers and witnesses in the midst of their trials.[10] The primary objection to this way of ordering the problem is that, by limiting God's power, it postulates a God unworthy of worship and no more or less useful to turn to in our difficulties than a compassionate friend.

Even a superficial review of different ways of approaching the "problem of evil," with their varying emphases, may help attune the ear of an attentive clinician—physician, nurse, chaplain—to common themes of suffering: guilt and punishment, growth and education, responsibility, isolation, and perplexity. As we try to aid patients and families in their struggle to find something good, something positive in what seems a thoroughly negative experience, we may learn to hear strains of the spiritual anxiety that can compound the injury. Many clinicians know the importance of receiving, and thus validating, the concerns of patients, whether they seem related to the unknowable consequences of an upcoming surgical procedure or to negotiating a present clouded by pain and a future dimmed by uncertainty. We seem, however, less able—or perhaps less willing—to recognize the deeper spiritual questions that may underlie some of these concerns: Where is God in all this? Why is this happening to me?

These sorts of questions also need validating reception, but they may require in addition more direct and specific attention. John Cobb has said:

> The pastor's task is to be present with the sufferer, to "hear" her or him, to let the parishioner know that the fear, anger, and loneliness that are felt can be expressed and will be accepted. I do not dispute the validity of this approach. In many cases it is no doubt the best possible.
>
> The question, Why?, can be appropriately understood and dealt with psychologically. But to treat it only that way is to fail to take the questioner with full seriousness as a human being. A pastor who has not reflected about the question, who has nothing to say, will have a truncated ministry.[11]

The same might be said of the medical practitioner receiving the plaintive questions that signal the work of theodicy in progress. It is not that doctors and nurses must be able to engage in religious discourse with patients. Rather, we can be prepared to recognize the spiritual import of such questions and grant them "full seriousness," a stance that may, at a minimum, give permission for the bold exploration to continue and, perhaps, suggest someone as a prepared guide for the journey.

This book is an attempt to show how those questions may be heard and what kinds of responses may or may not be appropriate. In the effort to work through that task, the chapters also give insight into various ways of understanding God's role in human suffering, with particular focus on the immediacy of the individual experience of medical affliction.

Pain Seeking Understanding

The opening chapter by *Larry D. Bouchard*, included in Part 1, "Clinical Perspectives," also serves as a prologue for the book. He explicates the distinction between the intellectual, abstract question of theodicy—the formal "problem of evil" and its capacity to impugn the justice, goodness, love, or power of God—and the practical anguish experienced in human instances of suffering and in human attempts to hear and help the sufferer. The reason for including this prologue in the opening part is this: Bouchard proposes that we avoid a search for comprehensive solutions, an enterprise that may deflect attention from the reality of acute need, and instead hold together whatever partial, fragmentary meanings and hopes we may possess in ways that can both consent to and resist pain, in the modes of recognition and lament characteristic of encounters with tragedy. Practical theodicy, then, begins from a clinical perspective.

The other four chapters in this part call upon clinical experience for observations about whether and how questions of theodicy arise, both for those suffering medical ills and for the health care professionals and clergy who attend to them, and about how such questions may be perceived and answered. *Deborah E. Healey*, a pediatrician and Christian layperson, presents stories from her practice, interlaced with meditations about the resources of faith available for her and for the children and families she sees. Her particular practice is such that she is confronted continually by material manifestations and consequences of moral evil, and her sense of the presence of God as goodness in the midst of that evil informs her practical theodicy.

In contrast, *Julia E. Connelly*, a general internist, is not a person of religious faith. Thus, instead of focusing on the presence or role of God, Dr. Connelly speaks of hearing and understanding the suffering of her patients; she invokes both the interpretive category of tragedy and the creation of poetry as means of grasping and ordering the incomprehensible nature of what she is trying to help heal. She demonstrates in her stories how a sensitive physician, although not herself a "believer," needs to be where her patients are, even as they struggle with God, in order to accompany them in their pain.

Albert H. Keller is a Protestant minister and ethicist whose career has largely entailed teaching and advising medical students and family medicine residents about their own spiritual needs and those of their patients. Here he presents a series of conversations with Drew, a parishioner who is also a physicist and father of a handicapped child. Through Drew's insights about chaos theory and intersections of indeterminacy, nonlinear causation, and responsibility, Keller makes salient points about seeking both truth and faithful ways of responding to suffering within the entanglements and patterns of our lives.

Following these three very different chapters, I—a pediatrician and theological ethicist—offer an analysis that ties them together, drawing out common descriptive and interpretive points about the nature of the theodicy question as it arises for and may be expressed by those seeking medical or pastoral care. The issues thus raised can then be construed in ways helpful to sufferer and professional alike, and the clinician may fashion fitting responses even in the absence of satisfactory answers.

Part 2 considers how traditional formulations of theodicy—in Roman Catholicism, Protestant Christianity, and Judaism—may speak to the problem of evil manifested in medical suffering. *Daniel P. Sulmasy*, a Roman Catholic (and a Franciscan) who is also a practitioner of internal medicine and a medical ethicist, puts forward a vigorous classical argument, based on the reality and pain of human finitude, for the logical plausibility of God's being both utterly good and omnipotent even in the face of real evil and suffering. Echoing Cobb's caution cited above, he claims an important role for such logical arguments in assisting sufferers to retain or regain their faith in and reliance on God's love and power, and thereby to transcend suffering that cannot be eliminated.

Wendy Farley, a Protestant Christian and a theologian, sets aside logical arguments like that offered by Sulmasy in favor of an insistence on God's goodness and presence, manifested as divine compassion. She wonders whether the traditional enterprise of theodicy might itself be evil, or in complicity with evil, because of its emphasis on guilt and desert, and postulates instead a theodicy that, along with the sufferer, seeks meaning and thereby resists evil. Repeating themes introduced by Bouchard, Farley speaks of the importance of embodiment and creation in God's image, emphasizing the need to hold together simultaneously the truths of human mortality and human beauty.

A summary of Jewish perspectives on health care and the dilemmas imposed by suffering is presented by *Elliot N. Dorff*, rabbi, ethicist, and philosopher of Judaism. His historically rich and concise review of Jewish theodicies reveals many similarities to Christian efforts to reconcile the apparently contradictory terms of the problem, and culminates in his own arguments for recognizing and appreciating God's presence in the good aspects of human life and for protesting God's accountability for evil. Having dealt with the scholastic question, he devotes a considerable portion of his chapter to practical responses to suffering suggested by Judaism.

Part 2 on theological perspectives ends with a chapter by *Per Anderson*, a Protestant Christian theologian and teacher. Anderson's work combines the concerns of the three preceding chapters by considering two "ideal types" of theodicy, the classical hermeneutical and the technological practical. Using the "Serenity Prayer" as his template, he argues for increased attention to traditional theodicies as a counterbalance to technology's assumption that everything can be fixed, an illusion that, Anderson believes, leaves us without the interpretive resources necessary for serenity despite unalterable suffering.

Part 3 has to do with implications and further questions arising from this study of "medical theodicy." Philosopher *James Lindemann Nelson* contributes an interesting twist on the subject of theodicy by identifying a *secular* problem of evil: the dilemma faced by those who want to act against the innumerable instances of injustice and suffering that are amenable to at least partial relief, but who also want to preserve for themselves adequate resources for the particulars that make their own lives meaningful and beautiful. After a thorough explication of this problem—including a defense of its reality and significance—Nelson postulates that the vocation of medicine may be a paradigmatic solution to the problem. Although he does not use theological or religious language, Nelson echoes what several other authors in this book claim about the importance of "doing" theodicy, of living out a resolution of the dilemmas of good and evil in creative and responsive action.

Ronald Cole-Turner, a Protestant theologian and ethicist, uses the tools of theodicy to work through questions about the existence of disordered gene sequences that may portend disease and suffering, seeking a theological interpretation and an appropriate pastoral response to questions about genetic testing and genetic "determinism." Much like the clinical chapters by Healey, Connelly, and Keller, Cole-Turner's chapter exemplifies the practical importance of theodicy questions as they arise in the context of painful choices, inescapable but confused lines of responsibility, and limited comprehension.

In addition to implications for the responsible clinician, the "problem of evil" as presented in these chapters also compels the attention of biomedical ethics. *Mark J. Hanson*, theological ethicist and associate of the Hastings Center, specifically addresses the significance of these discussions for rethinking the role and preoccupations of bioethics. After demonstrating that bioethics' (and medicine's) resources are insufficient to aid either practitioners or patients in their struggles to understand and handle suffering, he suggests that bioethics may serve more usefully as a "mediator" of resources from richer spiritual and moral traditions. In this he echoes the arguments of Anderson and others in this book for redirecting attention to the neglected value of accepting some suffering as unfixable, as tragic.

Hanson ends by listing six elements of an agenda that, if taken seriously by bioethics, could enable the discipline to mediate to sufferers and those who care for them the considerable resources of centuries of thought about evil, suffering, and divine intent and order. The book then concludes with an epilogue that recaps the themes of the chapters and briefly draws out similar implications for medical education, practice, and ethics.

Many years ago I led an adult church school class through a study of C. S. Lewis's lucid, compelling, and honest foray into theodicy, *The Problem of Pain*. We spent three months moving slowly through his arguments and our own remembered experiences of suffering. When we reached the end of the book, we agreed that we were no closer to an "answer" to the problem that evil poses for us as believers in a good and powerful God. But, we also agreed that somehow we were now much more content to leave the question unresolved, both because we had been brave enough to look it square in the face and because, by airing our bafflement and sharing our knowledge of evils suffered, we had taught each other many things about responding to suffering in the absence of a definitive answer. The editors and authors of this book hope that it will do something similar for its readers: expose the questions, display the nature and reality of the evil medicine sees as suffering, argue for and against an assortment of answers, and open new and rich ways of living with and responding to unanswerable questions and incomprehensible pain.

Part I

Clinical Perspectives

1

Holding Fragments

Larry D. Bouchard

Theodicy, it has been said, should be a practical and not only a theoretical issue.[1] Why practical? Perhaps because no theory, however reasonable, that reconciles God's ways with harm's way can insulate itself from the contradicting experiences of actual suffering. In such experiences, one's life—indeed one's world—is contradicted, shattered by *particular* harm. A practical theodicy should start with such particular expressions of tragic harm and contradiction. It may then set the fragmentary nature of harm, and any insights that may appear with such fragments, beside the fragmentary character of religious discernment. But to what effect? A practical theodicy must also, it seems, do something. Must it not in some way both *consent to* and yet *resist* harm? As I explore this question, I will suggest that a practical theodicy may consent and resist by "holding fragments": juxtaposing but not synthesizing fragmentary lives, traditions, and paths of thought.[2] I will juxtapose some odd passages of scripture, a play about a death from cancer, and a prayer for a cure for AIDS. And I will reflect on how "holding" them, without synthesizing them, may count as theodicy. The first fragments are from Luke, traditionally the disciple who was a physician.

At the site of the crucifixion, Jesus' mockers demand, "Save yourself!" In Luke one adds, "and us!" as well (23:39). Doctors remember another taunt. At synagogue, after proclaiming sight to the blind, Jesus also says, "Doubtless you will quote to me this proverb, 'Physician, heal yourself'" (4:23, RSV). This proverb is well known but of unknown origin. Absent its context, what can it mean? "Healing," sometimes, can connote "saving." Let us suppose an afflicted person speaks these words out of suffering as well as anger. Might they mean: "I'm not the one here who needs healing"? Or, "Don't touch me, you can't even heal yourself"? Or even, "Heal yourself, so you can heal me"? Or does the taunting proverb mean, paradoxically, "Save me!" though in disbelief that "I" can be saved?[3] Perhaps the new implication of the old proverb is that the physician should not turn inward, but should find a new way to turn outward, and also that issues of theodicy arise as much when medicine is perceived to fail as when God seems to fail.

13

Suffering and Evil as Concrete Experiences

In particular historical, social, and personal moments, we meet suffering and evil concretely. These moments seem intrinsically to demand that we, or someone, attend and act. Yet, while we encounter misfortunes concretely, we rarely encounter them simply—except, perhaps, in the immediacy of our own physical pain. Our own expressions of suffering, as well as the responses we offer to the suffering of others, are shaped and complicated by traditions—and not single traditions but many strands of many traditions. Even our outcries and our pained silences—indeed, our thinking, speaking, and ways of *feeling* in response to suffering—draw on historical currents of culture and language. They stream through our articulate and inarticulate gestures of pain, grief, and understanding.[4] As a teacher of religion, literature, and criticism, I myself am acquainted with four of these cultural currents: those of Greek tragedy and modern drama and those of the Bible and Christian thought. It is when the literary traditions of tragedy and the scriptural traditions jam together in our minds, like cool and warm air masses, that we enter the meteorology of the spirit called "theodicy." Theodicy can come of listening and speaking in at least two different yet compelling languages at once, those of tragic lament and biblical proclamation.

If we add another language to our encounters with suffering and evil, then we get our hybrid topic, "Theodicy and Medicine." For medicine is traditionary. It receives lore, values, and practices, which persist, change, and are handed on from master to apprentice, and from "insiders" to a wider public and culture. In the wider culture, its traditions mingle with both the literary and scriptural traditions. Concepts and "proverbs" of medicine enter common speech and shape our available language and perceptions of suffering. Medicine, in fact, may well be among the sources for contemporary theodicy.

Imagine a doctor who watches a patient, a mother's only child, die of a sudden, overwhelming infection. The mother says, "This must be God's will," believing with all the wisdom she can muster that God is taking her only child for some unknown but promised purpose. And the doctor, unable to cure, now struggles only to care and to refrain from saying, "No, God's power is not like that; God's goodness does not require this death," or else struggles not to say, "No! Your belief in such a meaningless God only compounds this pointless suffering." The doctor knows this is not the time for such remedial religious lessons. But for both the mother and the physician—who might also be a parent—the phenomenon, if we may call it that, of theodicy has transpired. A questioning word about justice and compassion that transcends suffering and evil has been thought, sought, or spoken.

But such questions may not exhaust the phenomenology of theodicy. Margaret Mohrmann, a pediatrician and ethicist, writes of being beside a widowed mother who, immediately upon her teenage son's death, began rocking in her chair by his bed. She wept, then mumbled, until she became articulate, able to ask, "Who's going to sit on the porch in the evening with me? Who's going to the grocery store with me?" Mohrmann realized, "I had no answer but my own tears."[5] Here the question is not one of transcendent justice, but of concrete meanings. Where am I now? What future can endow my mundane moments with meaning, after the reality of *this* death in *these* circumstances of *my* life? In the transition Mohrmann observed, from tears and murmurs to full, felt speech, the mother set out upon a new trajectory. She will speak, and her speech may elicit responses, which together will resist the void in which both speaker and hearer may for a long time find themselves. In the hybrid language I wish to explore, these responses—both the mother's query and the physician's silence, tears, and later testimony—are also moments when theodicy occurs.

I write as one skeptical of placing the language of theodicy adjacent to the language of pain and grief, that is, the language of tragic lament. My thinking is perhaps too hybrid. I am an irenic teacher of the fascinating "varieties of religious experience"; I am an ironic critic of culture and the arts; I am also a sometime freestyle theologian in an obscure though insistently "mainstream" Protestant denomination. My skepticism about theodicy originated in college and graduate school, when certain readings of Greek tragedy, existentialist theology, and Holocaust testimony led me to conclude that "solving" the "problem of evil" was deeply futile.

I am still skeptical, but perhaps more open to theodicy as well. For those who rail against theodicy are likely to be depending on it to fuel their negations and may be producing odd theodicies of their own. Moreover, if theodicy is a human concern before it is a theological topic, we cannot avoid it. Nonetheless, "doing" theodicy strikes me, at first, as rationalizing: an affair of forcing premises to fit the facts of history and nature and of explaining in universal terms how an omnicompetent Creator is not contradicted by the harms of the world. Not only classical theodicies (such as the free-will defense and the aesthetic harmony of good and evil) but even the most innovative "solutions"—such as those of process theology and contemporary views of "soul making"—seem only to be efforts to "save the face" of God rather than to discern the complications of suffering and evil.

As one reads or attends Greek and modern tragedies, one discovers testimonies of human *hubris*, fallibility, and violent anger—matters associated with culpability or moral evil. One also discovers testimonies of victims; of the relatively innocent who suffer at the whims of chance, society, nature; or of those for whom God and the world have become manifestly alien to human well-being. Tragic literature suggests that while moral evil and harmful contingencies are deeply distinguishable, in actual life they are also deeply entangled. In my parlance, "the tragic" refers to destructive *entanglements* of innocent contingency and moral culpability that play themselves out in different ways, in different stories, and in different lives.[6] To attend to the extreme outcries of people baffled by atrocity, or whose personal and familial worlds are darkened by illness or social affliction, is not merely to hear the projections of primitive religious distress, when they say that God has "struck them down" or "abandoned" them or is "testing" them. They can be, rather, the honest expressions of people whose horizons have foreclosed possibilities of flourishing, for whom the depths of themselves and of the world have erupted as a meaningless or destructive abyss.

Had the first mother said over her son that "this is God's will and God's will is wicked!" her witness would resonate with the laments of the elders in Aeschylus's *The Persians*, who hear news of the total destruction of their superior army. Had she wanted to say, "How pointless the world in which a mother survives a son," she might find phrases in Euripides' *Trojan Women*, as when Hecuba receives the corpse of her little boy, Astyanax. Or had she answered, "God has brought us to this horrible pass, yet I also am accountable," she would speak the language of *Oedipus the King*, marked by its extremity and severe self-scrutiny. A physician would be wrong to discount the meaning of these utterances and would be right to search attentively, carefully, and—as well—critically for their meanings.

But some, such as Paul Ricoeur and Martha Nussbaum, observe that religious and ethical thinking generally cannot abide such testimony. Coherent religious thought finds tragedy's disclosures of "malevolent transcendence," of "predestination to evil," or of "wicked gods" intolerable.[7] Ethics, likewise, has usually resisted tragedy's implication that one's being virtuous is contingent upon one's being lucky.[8] Faced with such testimonies of tragedy, thinking becomes cognitively dissonant and rationalizing. There may well be counter examples in which thought is able to tolerate such antinomian disclosures—especially if we grant that there is mythic and poetic as well as discursive reasoning.[9] But it is better to say that what resists religious and ethical thought is a sense of "rupture" in the tragic.

For instance, I may experience ethical rupture when I cannot separate the strands of moral evil and sheer contingency entwined in a tragic cord. As far as I trace them, I may find strands of both, but neither originates in the other. Moral evil and contingent harm are irreducible, but they complicate each other. Rupture may also appear when I sense that the very structures that sustain my life or my community now contradict it, and that wherever I turn there is no redemptive possibility of peace, rescue, or transformation. I might express this by lamenting that God—whom I formerly discerned as being with me—is now arrayed against me. I might demand with Job, "show me my fault," in order to make some sense of senseless harm. And while this sense of rupture might undermine the very basis for my religious thinking, such experiences of fearful transcendence do find fragmentary expression in religious witness. Psalm 88 is remarkable in that its lament that God is *against* the afflicted speaker is finally unmitigated by any hope that God will relent. It begins:

> O Lord, God of my salvation . . . let my prayer come before you; incline your ear to my cry.

After reviewing the torment of a despairing, isolated, unheard, and unremembered person nearing death, it ends:

> O Lord, why do you cast me off? Why do you hide your face from me? Wretched and close to death from my youth up, I suffer your terrors; I am desperate. Your wrath has swept over me; your dread assaults destroy me. They surround me like a flood all day long; from all sides they close in on me. You have caused friend and neighbor to shun me; my companions are in darkness.[10]

In ordinary times, few worshipers notice such complaints to God. But in times of great harm, they may transform as well as disturb us. For, roughly speaking, the Bible—and much of tragedy—counsels consent to the contingent nature of our lives, yet not consent to the point of resignation. Scripture counsels both consent and resistance in varying proportions, and both the consent and the resistance are further complicated by moral evil. Contingency and evil make us anxious; out of anxiety we may sin; sin may beget more sin and more contingent harm to ourselves and others; thus arises more anxiety.[11] Again roughly speaking, the Bible—and much of tragedy—counsels resistance against moral evil, yet not to the point of claiming false innocence nor of denying that moral dilemmas arise, accompanied neither by good choices nor by good answers. Lament, in both scripture and tragedy, can transform the reader in affirming that tragic rupture is both beyond our powers to control or comprehend and yet is to be resisted. Psalms of lament can offer us broken language when language is impossible. For Elie Wiesel, Emil Fackenheim, and others who reflect on language and faith after the Holocaust, such traditions provide ways to pray when God is manifestly absent, or ways to speak to the world when humanity is manifestly silent.[12]

The problems for theodicy raised by illness and medicine are not those of the Holocaust. The relentless, inexplicable policies of genocidal evil in Europe, and the kinds of suffering witnessed there, are not the contingencies of chronic illness, fatal accident, and epidemic, though moral evil complicates all of these. But it was Holocaust testimony that led me to listen for truth in the concrete, particular, and fragmentary witnesses of those who speak of irretrievable loss, or who say that God has abandoned them or that their trust in existence is "ruptured."[13] Such testimonies cause some to doubt the "good" of theodicy when it is set beside actual suffering and the limits of its comprehension. They have led

some Christians to hear in the last words of Jesus, as recorded in Mark and Matthew, a cry of abandonment that sets aside theodicy.

Theodicy as a Modern Problem?

One complaint about theodicy is that the "problems of evil" it addresses often
turn out to be problems of thought created by modern (i.e., post-seventeenth-
century) conceptions of God, nature, and the good. God, who in Western religious traditions is other than ourselves and transcends what reason can establish,
came to be viewed as something reason should explain comprehensively, or else
reject. But critics warn that inserting God into metaphysical or moral models of
reality that reject mystery only results in the "domestication" of transcendence,[14]
and can reflect historical-political patterns of power and enslavement. Be it God's
power or human power, for example, power is assumed to be only coercive, like
that of princes or police. Or goodness is assumed to be that of an impartial
magistrate who distributes rewards, penalties, and entitlements. Theodicy can
then become a kind of secular rationalization of the status quo,[15] or an exercise
in algebra, of the kind Voltaire satirized in the Leibnizian figure of Dr. Pangloss
in *Candide*. Pangloss explains how this orb of catastrophes is really "the best of all
possible worlds." In such algebra, it is more important to define and balance
God's power and goodness (on one side of the equation) with "bad things" (on
the other) than to confront concrete yet unquantifiable injustice, disease, grief,
and trauma—together with the particularities of justice, joy, and loving-kind-
ness—in the lives of persons and communities.

Alternatives to explanatory theodicies are religious visions that acknowledge
mystery and contradiction, from the perspectives of confessions, communities,
and critical practices. I am developing such a perspective here, but I must acknowledge discomfort with some criticisms of theology's "modern" heritage ("En-
lightenment-bashing" or "liberal-bashing" as it is sportingly called). First, I, like
all readers of this chapter, remain a child of modernity. Modern commitments to
critical science and to the values of political liberty and respect for persons ought
to be reexamined and qualified but hardly abandoned. Second, some "modern"
theologies are themselves modes of interpretive experience through which we
can encounter anew misfortune, injustice, and particular questions of God and
the world.

Post-Enlightenment theology offers some insights and principles that are not
hubris only, not webs of error only, but also gifts of which one may remain a
steward. As a postmodern child of modernity, I seek to think about God and
the world with both understanding and suspicion, in hermeneutical ways that
are critical of modernity's hubristic episodes. These are episodes of undervaluing

the traditionary character of understanding; of overvaluing individual autonomy; of slighting mythic, poetic, and aesthetic modes of knowing; and of ignoring the social and sexual plurality of humanity, as if modernity's own "enlightenment" were not itself traditionary, mytho-poetic, and plural. I certainly cannot enumerate all that is valuable in various modern theologies, through which we may encounter anew the tragic and gracious dimensions of the world. I will, however, risk naming a few principles that reflect certain modern retrievals of traditional limits on what we can say of God and the world (derived from more theologians than I know or can cite).[16] These axioms are heuristic, for the sake of discovery. They are not the most important things to be said here, and are not my conclusions. But they may clear some ground and, though densely summarized, may express something of what the first physician, above, could not say to the grieving mother yet wished to say, for the sake of both their integrities.

1. "No one has ever seen God" (John 1:18). God is discerned only through engaged responses to human testimonies about (and promises of) personal and world transformation. The testimonies are themselves also interpretive responses and anticipations. The histories of these discernments and responses are "religious traditions," and the sense of involvement they require is "faith." Western religious traditions speak of what is ultimately real and ethically required in an astonishing variety of media. The knowledge they disclose is "revealed," and its modes of disclosure are symbolic, narrative, dramatic, and analogical. In short, there is no neutral, uninvolved knowledge of God, only participatory and distinctively contextualized knowing.

2. Yet no expressions concerning God and the world are sufficient unto themselves, adequate to their aims, or complete in their relations of parts and wholes. All are partial and fragmentary, limited by (1) the infinity of God and the finitude of reason, (2) the contingent talents and strengths of people seeking to understand, and (3) the distortions of human interests and moral faults. The most discerning expressions of God and the world contain acknowledgments of their own inadequacy. They incorporate, albeit in partial ways, recognitions of the limits of experience and language when we are speaking of God. "I am a man of unclean lips," says Isaiah (6:5), as he describes how he was once indeed allowed to "see God."

3. In relating to the world, God is not a finite or "proximate" cause of particular events, such as this death or that birth. Jesus assured his disciples that God "sends rain on the just and the unjust" (Matthew 5:45). How or whether God conditions each drop is not discernible. Divine "grace" may well be the reason why particular lives and communities are transformed by possibilities of love and justice. Divine "immanence" may well mean that God is the indwelling source of meaning and novelty, of unanticipated possibilities within the spheres of humanity and nature. Divine "transcendence" may well mean that God is the "wholly

other" source and limit of the whole of reality. But God is not the immediate cause of this illness or that earthquake, this clinical depression, or that genocidal war—nor of this remission or that peace. God may be discerned *with* all actions and events or *within* them, as the power that enlivens them, the limit that negates them, and the infinity that recalls them. God, in short, is the reality that limits all reality and gives more reality.

4. "Neither are your ways my ways, says the Lord" (Isaiah 55:8). And "My kingdom is not of this world," Jesus tells Pilate (John 18:36). To speak of God's "power" is to speak symbolically and analogically, in terms of our experiences of power: political, personal, and natural. However, because "power" terms ascribed to God are figurative and because God is infinite and other, it should be said that God's power is unlike human and natural power structures. God's is not the power of a parliament or corporation, not the power of a magnetic personality or a quiet teacher, not the power of a tide or a heartbeat. Rather, God may be discerned in figures opposed to worldly power: divine power as the powerlessness of a child or a prisoner, wisdom as human folly, wealth as poverty, identity as self-loss, sovereignty as exile, presence as absence. God may be discerned when our "idealism" is disappointed or transformed or, conversely, when our "realism" about life and political power is challenged.

5. Because forms of love (e.g., parental love, friendship, erotic desire and joy, love of justice, of knowledge, of nature, and of beauty) provide profound analogies for God, we may discern God in acts of love. Nonetheless, God-as-love is other than human loves. When God "so loves the world" (John 3:16), it is not a general love that dissolves particularity; and when God loves in particular, as "When Israel was a child I loved him and out of Egypt I called my son" (Hosea 11:1), the particularity of such loving, calling, or electing does not exclude the world. The implication is not so much that God's love is the perfection of human love, but that God's love sometimes illuminates and sometimes contrasts with how humans love.

While these axioms might seem to be the components of an explanatory theodicy, I do not regard them so. It is true, they do qualify God's power and goodness, and so they might lessen the burden of theodicy by appealing to divine mystery and the limits of human understanding. But in affirming that God, while other than ourselves, is discerned *within* our relations with others and with nature—thus implying that God is not so "wholly other"—these axioms may make theodicy more, not less, painful to contemplate. For they do not soften the implication that God must inhere in both beauty and horror. They neither insulate God from actual evil and suffering nor absolve God's accountability as the Other whose participation, or whose absence, may or may not be discerned in any realities and possibilities.

Elements of a Practical Theodicy

Minimally, a practical theodicy understands suffering and evil by resisting the effects or consequences of suffering and evil. There is, implicitly, something of practical as well as cognitive resistance in the very phenomenon of theodicy. When the first mother said, "This must be God's will," she may or may not have been stating a settled, considered conviction. But certainly she was resisting purposelessness and pain, in behalf of her son, herself, and perhaps others—such as the physician. We do not know, immediately, how to assess her statement. Is she denying a truth, that life is filled with unjustifiable harm; or is she resisting a counsel of despair, that unjustifiable harm empties all life of extraordinary goods and meanings? We do not know the consequences of her resistance: will it knit wounds or open new ones?

Likewise, when the first physician thinks, "No, God's power is not like that; God's goodness does not require this death," or "No! Your belief in such a meaningless God only compounds this pointless suffering," resistance is also occurring. How shall we assess it? Is the doctor railing against illusion, against justifying the unjustifiable, against dissolving into platitude the particularity of this son's death and this mother's loss? Or is the doctor's own helplessness more at stake? Does the doctor's silent protest aim to understand the mother's travail, or to keep the doctor insulated from her grief? Could it not be all these things? In any case, the doctor implies that some ideas, when pursued to logical conclusions, do particular harm; so to resist them is to resist harm.

Thus a paradox emerges: If I rail against theodicy, then my railing is itself a way to resist suffering and evil; and by resisting them, I set them in a particular place of encounter that is no longer so meaningless. By resisting the consequences of certain, perhaps totalizing, ideas about suffering and evil, I can at least bring to a particular place of encounter the fragmentary meanings of my life or the lives I share. My protest can become a practical theodicy that refuses sheer harm as the last thing to be said of these lives or of creation. In respect to theodicy, I may resist the idea that "the tragic" is metaphysically final, and yet refuse to finally explain those places and moments where life, language, and thought have been utterly, despairingly broken. To so resist and to so refuse together define an act of loving compassion and moral urgency.

The meanings we bring will be fragmentary, not complete meanings. Why fragmentary? Because harm is fragmenting, and we are fragmentary. We are historical beings, and each of us hails not from one but from many traditions with deep currents of language, stories, and images. We are, moreover, embodied, both organically and culturally. Each of us is an integral whole, but none is completely whole. None of us is as strong, clever, or wise as we might be. None of us can experience enough, in our one life, to know what we need to know, or feel what there is to feel. None, throughout our lives and from moment to moment, is as virtuous as we might be. None of us can live long on our own, yet we all do our own dying. The world we encounter is whole and fragmentary—both generally and in utterly particular, novel ways. Consequently, we live and understand only as we receive and pass on fragmentary meanings from other lives, be these mean-ings gifts, burdens, or curses to ourselves.

Thus, one approach to practical theodicy will be the juxtaposing of partial meanings.[17] Here, motifs of tragic lament and prayers of protest are set beside witnesses to God's own suffering, which in turn abut with pleas that hold God accountable to suffering. Juxtaposition is an alternative to positing a total frame-work of thought. By "holding fragments," I do not mean being irrational, for to think with the fragments requires critical reasoning and assessment. (We may ask, whence these fragments? How are they appropriate to this encounter or these issues?) But I do mean to leave incomplete the bridges of thought between the stories, images, or actions we juxtapose. What now traverses the distance be-tween the fragments may simply be the living, working, and abiding with others, even in the distances that separate us. What crosses between lamentation, soli-darity, and protest may be attentive silence, or the recital of a psalm, or—as here—the stories of those who have also held fragments. Minimally, by holding shards of life and meaning, by juxtaposing but not synthesizing them, we decide that in "this matter," or at "this time and place," we leave further, connective explanation to others and for another time. Maximally, we open a space in which redemptive possibilities may, or may not, later appear.

No Shadows and Only Shadows

Those familiar with the life of C. S. Lewis know that after he married Joy Davidman his views on love began changing, and that upon her death from cancer he expe-rienced a severe crisis of faith. This rupture is recorded in his memoir, A *Grief Observed*, and in three versions of *Shadowlands* (a TV drama, then a stage play, later a film). Since the film has made the gist of the story widely known, I will only comment on moments from the stage version by William Nicholson,[18] in which Lewis can be said to "juxtapose fragments." Early on, he delivers a popular talk, referring to a bus crash that killed twenty-three children. He asks why a loving God didn't stop it. His tone is confident, certain of his argument, which justifies pain by its spiritual benefits. "I think that God doesn't necessarily want us to be happy. I think He wants us to be lovable. Worthy of him. Able to be loved by him." God creates us free to be loving or selfish, and selfishness makes us hard to love. So God has also created a "mechanism"—pain and suffering—

"which will penetrate our selfishness and wake us" from our "dream that all is well," from our illusions of "self-sufficiency."

> God loves us, so he makes us the gift of suffering. Through suffering, we release our hold on the toys of this world, and know that our true good lies in another world.
>
> We're like blocks of stone, out of which the sculptor carves the forms of men. The blows of His chisel, which hurt so much, are what make us perfect. The suffering in the world is not the failure of God's love for us; it is that love in action.
>
> For believe me, this world that seems to us so substantial, is no more than the shadowlands. Real life has not begun yet.[19]

At the beginning of Act II, after the onset of Joy's cancer, Lewis delivers a similar talk. But the tone is no longer so bracing. The particular, "real life" realities of his growing love for Joy, and his helplessness before her pain, bring out implications he senses are intolerable. "I find it hard to believe that God loves her," he says, intending to be merely rhetorical. "If you love someone, you don't want them to suffer. You can't bear it. You want to take their suffering on to yourself. If even I feel like that, why doesn't God?" He repeats that the sculptor-God offers "the blows of his chisel" to perfect us, to awaken us from our illusions. But in the midst of this trope, Lewis interrupts himself to ask, "But after they have suffered, must they still suffer more? And more?" The stage direction says he has no answer; he can only "repeat his familiar lines, wanting to believe them."[20]

Lewis and Joy receive the sacrament of marriage at what seems to be her deathbed. Yet her cancer remits, and they spend three idyllic years together, a happiness that ruptures Lewis's former views as much as did her cancer. They know the disease will someday recur, and so Joy offers a new theodicy: the "pain [to come] is part of this happiness, now. That's the deal."[21] When she does die, Lewis is shattered. In *A Grief Observed*, he says he did at last recover and move from near paralyzing grief to a different mode of faith.[22] Nicholson dramatizes this "recovery" in a speech that is both resilient and contradictory, in the sense that fragmentary tropes are allowed to stand in tension without resolution. Lewis returns to the sculpting image: "We are blocks of stone . . ." That the one who chisels is "God" is implied, but could just as easily be "life." Then a pause and a different thought: "No shadows here"—meaning either that Lewis is under no illusions, or that this life is not illusory but altogether real.

> No shadows here. Only darkness, and silence, and the pain that cries like a child. It ends, like all affairs of the heart, with exhaustion. Only so much pain is possible. Then, rest.
>
> So it comes about that, when I am quiet, when I am quiet, she returns to me. There she is, in my mind, in my memory, coming towards me and I love her again as I did before, even though I know I will lose her again, and be hurt again.
>
> So you can say if you like that Jack Lewis has no answer to the question after all,

except this: I have been given the choice twice in my life. The boy chose safety.
The man chooses suffering.

The pain, now, is part of the happiness, then. That's the deal.

Only shadows, Joy.[23]

Between "no shadows" and "only shadows," I suggest, is nothing more logical,
nor less, than the particularities of two lives lived in passion, pain, and long-
remembered conversation. Lewis now leaves others to make discursive connections between the fragments. His "no shadows/only shadows" is still theodicy,
centered on the idea of choosing suffering: if you are offered love and suffering,
choose not the illusion of safety (by living in isolation) but choose what you are
given. For only by such choice, by claiming a given love and a given pain, is
happiness possible. His practical theodicy is born of grief and resists despair. By
implication, it resists the threat of despair to others (such as to Joy's son, Douglas,
whom I have not discussed). And its urgent axioms—"the pain, now, is part of
the happiness, then"; "the boy chose safety, the adult chooses suffering"—do
indeed address real questions, for some inquirers, at some painful times. But these
axioms, too, are liable to rupture, if one day we come to confess that no happiness *then* coheres with *this* pain now, nor can *this* resurrection of happiness now
justify *that* pain then. One can imagine a moment when the admonition, "choose
the suffering, make it your own," would seem but resignation, not active resistance. The alternative, then, might well be to shout, "No! We do not accept this
suffering, this happy hammer-blow of God! Nor should you!"

This response, a kind of protest toward God, is apparently more familiar to
Judaism than to Christianity. It is a protest often made in behalf of communal
rather than individual suffering, though both Psalm 88 and the speeches of Job
are spoken by afflicted, solitary persons. In Judaism, the focus of redemptive concern is corporate: the people Israel. So prayers of protest and argument are addressed to God in behalf of the community. Wiesel describes a scene in Auschwitz
in which God was put on trial, found guilty, then prayed to. He writes of messen-
gers carrying protests *to* God, rather than *from* God.[24] Such prayers afford ways to
remain in dialogue with God when communion has been broken off, seemingly
by God's silence and humanity's silence. Such prayers hold God to account and
hold God's promises in tension with present catastrophe. They say in effect, "God,
be God!"—as if to awaken God from slumber, so as to attend to these matters at
this time.

Tony Kushner, playwright of *Angels in America*, delivered such a prayer at the
1994 Episcopal National Day of Prayer for AIDS, in the Church of St. John the
Divine in New York City. Kushner's religious vision is inseparable from his political vision. God, if at all affirmed in the play, is to be discerned in the solidarity of
the suffering and the dying with life. One woman in *Angels*, Harper, envisions
the souls of the dead rising in rings of three—as if three atoms of oxygen—to

heal the hole in the ozone layer. Here, I am less concerned with Kushner's "the-ology" (apocalyptic? pantheistic? liberationist?) than with how the form and meanings of his AIDS prayer, a petitionary prayer to arouse an indifferent God, seek to effect something of what they petition.

"God:" he begins. "A cure would be nice."[25]

Parody is held in tension with urgency—*parody* because the prayer spoofs those who believe that God sends or deigns to alleviate specific episodes of trauma; *urgency* because each petition is prophetic, compassionately demanding that each terror afflicting each group or person—both the wise and the foolish, the just and the unjust—be resisted, immediately. In the first third of the seven-page prayer, the petitions proliferate and cascade on behalf of more and more people, in lists that read like catalogues of the tormented and the tormentors.

> Reconstitute the shattered. . . . Return to the cattle, the swine and the birds the intestinal parasite, the invader of lungs, the eye-blinder, the brain-devourer, the detacher of retinas. Rid even the cattle and the birds of these terrors; heal the whole world. Now. Now. Now. Now.
>
> . . . Protect: the injection drug user, the baby with AIDS, the sex worker, the woman whose lover was infected, the gay man whose lover was infected; protect the infected lover, protect the casual contact, the one-night stand, the pickup, the put-down, protect the fools who don't protect themselves, who don't protect oth-ers: YOU protect them. The misguided, too, and the misinformed, the ambivalent about living, show them life, not death. . . .
>
> Even John O'Connor, even Bob Dole, Giuliani and Gingrich, Jesse Helms and Pat Robertson—tear open their hearts, let them burn with compassion, stun them with understanding, ravish their violent, politick, cynical souls, make them wiser, better, braver people. You can. You, after all, are God. This is not too much to ask.

After this cascade of petitions, the hectoring tone turns reflective, alternating between interrogative and declarative. "Must grace fall so unevenly on the earth?" "Your silence, I must tell you . . . is outrageous." "Is prayer," as at the Wailing Wall, "mere attrition, a kind of endurance?" Kushner then takes up the mode of narrative, juxtaposing a tale of a Hasidic master, who futilely begged God to send the Messiah, with a clipping about a boy who refused to follow his beckoning AIDS mother into the Hudson, where she drowned. "What's become of the child of Milagros Martinez? Where is he now? . . . [W]hat river courses through his dreams at night . . . toward what conceivable future?"

Near the close, the petitions do seem extravagant. Though "in the habit of asking small things of you," Kushner now demands cures for everything, from breast cancer to capitalism to the restoration of the dead, including his mother. "Or at least guarantee that loss is not irrecoverable, so that life can be endured." While schooled in atheism, now "I almost know you are there. I think you are our home." "You have left bread-crumb traces inside me. Rapacious birds swoop

down and the traces are obscured, but the path is recoverable. It can be discovered again." His strategy has been to shout so outrageously as to awaken God, the
dead, and those who overhear the shouting—those who worsened the pandemic
by infected speech or inhuman silence, and especially those in whose behalf
Kushner, a survivor "by accident," shouts. Who can say what discerning and
enduring and healing effects are not accomplished by his exhortation? The last
petition is for human time.

> If you cannot do these things for us, we will do them for ourselves, but slowly,
> because we can't see far ahead. At least give us the time to accomplish the future.
> We had a pact; you engendered us.

We may ask, what effect can petitionary prayers of any kind have on the Creator
of the whole of proximate causes but of no cause in particular? The answer, in
this prayer, is that by calling God to account we are exposed to the divinely
created depths of our own accountability. We reassert the covenant between
God and Noah in the opposite direction. If you, O God, will not or cannot, we
will; for so you have made us—left such "bread-crumb traces" in us—that we will
attempt to keep your fractured promises.

Practical theodicy will authorize the afflicted to call God into account and yet
also attend to the promise of God's solidarity with affliction. I see no way, however, to think coherently about a "fit" between these fragments: one that says
God transforms irrecoverable loss through solidarity with the lost (as when God
goes into exile with the exiled or is forsaken with the God-forsaken) and another
that is compelled to speak into the capricious silence of God, and thus hold God
to holy account. The New Testament is itself based on a juxtaposition of incommensurate fragments: Crucifixion / Resurrection, God is dead / God is raised. But
its proclamations do not provide paradigms of protest so readily as do the Hebrew
Scriptures, in which God is aroused by the community to resume, as it were,
creative and providential resistance against primordial chaos.[26] So one must ask,
is there a scriptural basis for the Church to demand that God be God, and yet
affirm that God is radically at one with the suffering of creation?

In the first three Gospels there is the motif of Jesus' mockers, who protest that
if he is the Son of God, let him come down from the cross and save himself.[27]
Their protest is ironic if the reader believes the cross saves. There is also the
motif of God-forsakenness (in Mark and Matthew), in which Jesus dies uttering
the first lines of the lament in Psalm 22, "My God, my God, why have you forsaken me?" In the trinitarian interpretation of Jürgen Moltmann, this moment
may be seen as God being abandoned even by God. Thus, death in despair does
not trump God; God, by undergoing despairing death, "cries with and intercedes
for" those abandoned in such death.[28] Even radical nothingness cannot overcome God's outpouring in kenotic love (as in Romans 8:35–39).

Perhaps neither of these fragments, protest or shared forsakenness, is alone sufficient. Only to protest, "God, be God!" might leave us merely waiting, as if for Godot. And only to affirm God's own God-forsakenness may not account for, or "justify," the despair of irreparable harm and loss; that is, God-forsakenness and resurrection may "comprehend" yet still not "justify" the God-forsaken of the world. After Auschwitz, warns Fackenheim, to "stake all on divine power-lessness" implies Jews would have to become Christians.[29] And to anyone despairing of utter loss, the cross and the Resurrection without the angry or hopeless petitions of the afflicted might imply that on the cross God does not in fact comprehend all suffering and hopelessness.

To hold both fragments means valorizing Christ's mockers, something that, to my knowledge, Christian exegetes never do. Yet not to valorize them would be to forget that God surely holds their suffering too, an idea that is at least authorized by the first words from the cross in Luke. Christ prays, "Father forgive them; for they do not know what they are doing" (although this text is not found in all the early texts; hence, it is a fragment). What must God's "solidarity" include? Surely judgment and forgiveness and infinite compassion. And who are the mockers? They are the religious authorities, the chief priests and scribes, the "elders" (Matthew), and "rulers" (Luke). They are Roman soldiers who robed and "crowned" him "King of the Jews." They are the unspecified "bystanders" and in Luke include one of the thieves also crucified. Jesus is mocked by everyone except the male disciples (who have abandoned him) and three women (who have not). How do they mock? In Mark and Matthew, the bystanders wag their heads and say that he who would raze and rebuild the temple in three days should save himself and come down from the cross. The priests and scribes and, in Luke, the rulers say, "He saved others; let him save himself, if he is the Messiah of God, his chosen one." And also in Luke the first thief asked, from his cross, "Are you not the Messiah? Save yourself and us!"

What Christians must imagine, to hold these fragments, is that the authorities, the bystanders, the thief, and at least one soldier (who later calls Christ "a son of God," or "innocent") all mock him not only out of sin, but also out of suffering. They who have awaited deliverance are impatient with God; they say more than they know when they demand, "save yourself . . . and us as well!" They—whose country is occupied by imperial Rome, which will soon scour the land of Jews and destroy the temple—speak not only in unaccountable malice but also out of accountable woe. When they cry, "save yourself, save us," there is the sense, I suggest, they are holding God to account. It is true that in Luke the second criminal pronounces judgment upon the first and upon himself: "We indeed have been condemned justly." But when he asks to be remembered, "when you come into your Kingdom," he may share the expectation that the Messiah will come as a mighty ruler. If so, he misunderstands just as others have, and so mocks unwittingly, yet he is accepted with Christ "today . . . in Paradise." So when Christ says, "Why have you forsaken me?" and "Father, forgive them," he accepts their accountability as God's own accountability, and transforms their mockery into laments and petitions.

The story of the mockers demands that God be God. The story of Christ's abandonment holds and authorizes, in compassion, the demand of the mockers. This circle is not vicious. It is an expanding circle of memory and care—a "pouring out," or *kenosis* (Philippians 2:7–8)—in the midst of perplexity, hatred, and despair. It is a spinning outward into the hopeless and the hopeful. To the question of justifying the ways of God in times of harm, the practical answer is to hold humanity and God to account and attempt to heal oneself by healing others and demanding, awaiting, and discerning in urgent hope the healing of another.[30]

2

Painful Stories, Moments of Grace

Deborah E. Healey

I am a pediatrician in a university teaching hospital, on the faculty of a medical school. As is true for many others in such positions, my job description is like a large and leaky umbrella that protects me in some ways but also leaves me vulnerable to a wide variety of professional demands. My usual clinical work is with outpatients in a general pediatric clinic and in a teen health clinic. In these settings, I see children for well checks and acute illnesses. I provide comprehensive care and reproductive services for adolescents, and serve as a consultant in child sexual abuse. Both of the outpatient clinics where I work serve predominantly low-income families and individuals, many of whom struggle with constant economic hardship and tremendous daily demands. Often they tell me stories of misery and suffering that sometimes seem overwhelming. My medical care of these patients may be couched in terms of diseases and medicines, but it encompasses much more than the rudiments of treatment I was taught in medical school. At times, my whole being is drawn into hearing and receiving the stories, and I call on everything I know to help move my patients toward healing.

This chapter contains the stories of patients I have cared for during my years of medical practice. I am grateful for their trust and openness in telling me about their lives. To honor their confidence in me, I have changed their names and altered any identifying details. Some stories are composites drawn from the histories of several patients. Thus, what I relate is fiction that tells the truth about the suffering I see.

I am aware of God's presence in my work in several ways. My patients or their parents may talk about their illnesses or other afflictions in terms of their understanding of who God is. When that is how the illness is perceived, to hear and intervene I must use the same language, the same frame of reference. A recent patient encounter is a good example of this. A young adolescent girl was referred to me from her school psychologist. Over the past few months she had become quite withdrawn and depressed, spending hours alone in her bedroom curled up under the covers in the dark. Every day she vomited after each meal, and she declared to me that she felt fat. Her parents were deeply concerned about her and at a loss to understand what was wrong.

Clearly this was a complex situation, likely to include a mixture of old and new issues. At subsequent visits, I began to understand some of the stresses that this child was dealing with, most recently having to keep secret from her parents her older brother's drug use. I got the sense that she had lost her voice in this family and felt completely ineffective, with no way to express herself. She could live up to her family's expectations of her from the outside, but was powerless to know herself from the inside. My medical intervention included a number of recommendations and suggestions; I did not initiate antidepressant medication at first but elected to wait until she had begun in psychotherapy.

Some weeks later, she was dramatically improved and no longer depressed. There had been a real turnaround. I asked her what had made the difference for her. After a few moments, she quietly responded, "My faith." I was interested in her sense of God's role in her recovery. She told me that they had done this together, that God was working with her. We reviewed the specific changes she had been able to make. She knew how to recognize if things were not going so well again, and what she would need to do to get back on track. I told her that I could honor the importance of her faith in God.

Other families tell me of God's goodness. Mandy is seventeen and is moderately retarded and wheelchair-bound by her cerebral palsy. Her family lives some hours away in rural Virginia. Recently their old frame house burned down in an electrical storm. The dry wood burned fast, and the house was completely destroyed. The family told me, "God was looking out for us." Mandy's mother had been away with their older daughter, who had just had her first baby. During her mother's absence, Mandy and her father stayed with other relatives, so no one had been home at the time of the fire. The family was rejoicing: "It could have been so much worse; someone could have died." I have no doubt that this family's unshakable belief in God's goodness has much to do with the positive way they have been able to cope with the challenges presented by Mandy's illness and day-to-day care. I see how their faith empowers them to interpret their lives and to take action when needed, with confidence. To build on their strengths is a pleasure for me.

Sometimes in my work I hear concepts of God and God's will that are far from my own beliefs. Susie was eighteen; she had graduated from a small Christian high school and had the opportunity to go away to college. This was what her mother dearly wanted for her. Susie's mother had devoted enormous amounts of energy to giving Susie the best of everything throughout her childhood. Her own life had not been easy. There had been several unsuccessful marriages, at least one destroyed by alcoholism. Susie's older brother was seriously impaired by drinking and at that time was unemployed, still living in the family home. Susie had been able to grow through her adolescence, finding some sort of balance between who she was and who her mother wanted her to be. But now Susie's period was several weeks late and her pregnancy test was positive. She was thrilled and so happy; her mother was devastated. I talked privately with Susie's mother, who asked, "How have I failed? Look how much I did for Susie. What could I have done differently?" She told me that she prayed that Susie would miscarry, and urged me to encourage Susie to terminate the pregnancy. Abortion is not something she approves of, but under the circumstances . . .

Part of Susie's mother's distress turned out to be related to the fact that Susie had been dating a young man who is African American. Her family is Caucasian and not tolerant of racial difference. While I could hear the intensity of the mother's anguish, I could not share her prayer, and I could not do as she asked. I cannot encourage a patient to end a pregnancy; I can only guide her through the decisions she faces and support the choice she makes. I also realize that in my own prayers I find it difficult to make specific requests of God. I ask more that I might know God's purpose, that at any given time of stress I may have the discernment to know God's will and the strength to carry it out.

To return to the story, in this case the mother was not my patient; Susie was. I could hear the mother's distress and acknowledge it, but I could not ease it as she wanted me to. I had known them both for some years and had frequently talked with each of them about the good and the not-so-good events and challenges in Susie's life that they have had to face. Susie was my patient, she was no longer a minor, and she was rejoicing in the new pregnancy. Contrary to her mother's wishes, I shared her happiness, saying that I was delighted for her. Later, when the baby was born, Susie's mother fell in love with him on sight and became a doting grandmother with photos on hand to share with all. I have not asked her if she thinks God's will was done, though I imagine she would smile and say that it was.

More often, my patients talk about God at times when their own suffering seems unbearable to them. I recall a family in which there was a concern of possible child molestation, based on some disturbing comments made by the child. I was asked to evaluate her for any physical signs consistent with child sexual abuse. Crystal was four, and had already had serious medical problems with a cancer in one eye. The diseased eye had been removed and, as part of her follow-up care, her healthy eye had to be examined carefully, under anesthesia, every six months to make sure that it remained cancer-free. As there were no ongoing concerns for Crystal's safety, I agreed to combine her assessment with her next routine eye check, so that she could be asleep.

The time came, and I met first with Crystal's mother and aunt, who were still quite distraught about the possibility that Crystal had been sexually abused. When I examined the child, to my astonishment I could find no vaginal opening. The tissues all seemed healthy; the other openings were there as expected, but she had no genital outlet. This is an uncommon anatomical oddity, in no way related to childhood cancers or to abuse. I returned to the family and embarked on explaining my findings. First, there was no physical evidence to confirm their worry about abuse. This did not mean that we could prove it had not happened, but for further information we would have to go back to the comments Crystal had made, and try to understand what she had been telling them. Second, I had found something completely unexpected that we needed to discuss in detail and that would require more evaluation.

"How can God do this to a child?" they asked me when they heard this news. I can provide no answer to that question. But I can receive from them their confusion, their fears for Crystal and her future, their sense of helplessness and lack of control, even their anger at Crystal's having yet another problem to live with. I can help bear their burden. I guide them on to sort out what must happen next, and what will be asked of Crystal. They do not need to deal with this alone. I am there to help them through. I try to find some grain of hope to strengthen them.

Recently I took care of another girl—I shall call her Ann—who taught me something different about what faith can mean. Ann is fourteen, an eighth-grader from a rural county in the mountains. She had just disclosed to her mother that she had been raped two days earlier. The police were already involved and Ann had been examined by a local doctor, who reported evidence of forced vaginal penetration. As an expert in both adolescent medicine and child sexual abuse, I was asked to confirm the findings. I met with Ann alone. The story was quite straightforward: Ann had been at the home of Beth, another eighth-grader, and the two of them went to meet two young men at a motel. These men were both about nineteen; one of them was Beth's boyfriend. Beth and her boyfriend had sex. Although urged by Beth to have sex with the other man, Ann refused. She was then raped by him.

When I first met Ann, she was in the examining room by herself, sitting at the end of the exam table. I introduced myself, touched her gently on her shoulder, and asked her how she was doing. She burst into tears and said, "I feel terrible." Then she told me that she felt so ashamed: "I've let my mom down." Later in our conversation I introduced the idea of therapy, and went back to what she had told me about feeling terrible. Just how bad had she felt? She said that she had wanted to die. Had she thought about how that might happen? Had she made a plan? She then said, "I just asked God to let me die; I asked him to take me." My questions had come from the need to discern any potential risk of suicide; she answered me from her heart. With some hesitation, not quite knowing how she might take it, I pressed her a little, asking her how she thought God had responded to her request. With a quiet but steady voice, she said, "I guess he wanted me to stay with my mom." Her certainty in her faith was powerful.

When I spoke with Ann's mother at the close of the visit, I asked what part faith played in their lives. I wanted to find out whether Ann's turning to God, and her reliance on what she believed to be God's will for her, would be reinforced and supported by her family. I found that they had been regular churchgoers, but not for the past two years since the previous preacher left. Ann's mother had heard good things about the current preacher and had been thinking of returning to the church. With Ann's permission I shared with her Ann's comments to me about her faith, and encouraged her to make the reconnection with church as one of the concrete ways that she could help her daughter through what had happened and through the stress of the investigation to come.

Teaching what I know to medical students and young doctors is a large part of my daily work. Much of what I hear from my patients and their families and learn from the physical examination has enormous emotional content. We, as professionals, need first to care for the patients. But we also have to cope with our own responses to their situations. After ten years of doing this work I am in no way used to hearing the stories, and I have not become numb to my patients' pain. It is quite the contrary. I feel very directly for them and believe that, in order to provide compassionate care, I must be open to hearing just how bad things have been. Becoming numb might protect me in the short term, but it would also prevent me from forming any intimate connection with the family. I must be touched by the stories if I am to be an effective physician. Then, in order to care for myself I must recognize the basis of my reactions and deal with them in healthy ways that both heal me and allow me to see the next patient, to hear the next story. I try to teach our trainees these self-care coping skills along with the medical content of our patient encounters. I help them identify their own reactions to patients and what they might now do with them. With whom might they expect to share the story? What will that person then do with the information, particularly if he or she is not a medical professional? What about patient confidentiality? Has this story raised any particular issues from the past for the trainee?

I recall very clearly a first-year resident whom I already knew from having taught her when she was a medical student. I was now enjoying seeing her develop her clinical skills as a primary care doctor. Together we evaluated a three-year-old child, whom I shall call Wanda, for the possibility of sexual abuse. The story was troubling. Wanda had always slept in her parents' bed, as is not uncommon in our patient population. Since the birth of a second child eighteen months previously, the mother had taken to sleeping with the baby, while Wanda continued to sleep in the parental bed with her father. For the past two months, she had become increasingly passive and withdrawn, and she was now refusing to sleep with her father. At times, Wanda spoke what her mother described as "gibberish," nonsensical speech. We heard examples of this speech during the interview. Wanda did some normal age-appropriate talking, but after a few remarks she launched into unintelligible vocalizations that included the lilting expressions and even the nonverbal gestures of apparently meaningful communication.

Her physical examination showed us clear evidence of vaginal penetration and indications of repeated anal penetration. I was aware of my mouth stiffening as I completed the exam. This has long been a way I impose physical control on myself and has become a signal alerting me to some particularly challenging demand—in this case, the horror of realizing what this child had experienced. Perhaps most disturbing to me was her behavior. When I told Wanda that I needed to "check her pee hole and her poop hole," she immediately lay back completely limp and closed her eyes, with no expression on her face. She stayed like this, despite my efforts to reengage her, until I said that we had finished. She then reverted to the child I had seen earlier, quiet but interactive and present. The resident and I finished our session with the family and walked back to our work area.

I needed to debrief the resident, to help her release some of her emotions connected to this encounter. I also needed to deal with my own emotional response, my stiff mouth. I wanted to help this young doctor identify how she could move beyond the immediate impact of the horror to comprehend her responses and find some way to integrate this experience into her professional self, neither denying nor ignoring her reactions but being prepared to recognize them when they arise again in her work, and possibly even drawing on them to help her patients. When I asked her how she felt about what we had just been through and how she might be able to deal with it, she said with assurance, "I pray to God for the child; I pray for the mother." Then, with some real doubt in her voice, "But I'm finding it difficult to pray for the father." We talked of suffering and of pain. I told her my own solution, which is to offer up to God the entire situation, rather than specific individuals or pieces of the whole. I cannot begin to fathom these things alone. Not only is it impossible for me to understand how anyone can treat a child in such a way, but I also cannot bear the knowledge of it, of what I have observed in Wanda and my fears for her future. How psychologically damaged is she? How much healing is possible? Can her mother provide her with what she needs? I was very angry; even now, revisiting the story as I write this, all my emotions from that encounter return in full force. The whole situation is a real burden that I have inadequate resources to carry alone. I must give it to God in order to go on.

This story clearly raises the issue of my being confronted with evil in my work. There is no doubt that what happened to Wanda is evil, by any definition of the word. To reflect further on this, I need to recount another situation, again involving abuse. A four-year-old boy and his three-year-old sister were in foster care after concerns arose that they may have been abused and neglected by their family. Each child had disclosed physical abuse. They talked of having been thrown down stairs and out of windows, deprived of food and water, forced to eat feces and drink urine. They also alleged sexual abuse, involving penetration of every possible orifice. Multiple abusers were named, including both parents and two of the mother's boyfriends. I heard from the social worker that their mother would sit on the children's heads and urinate into their mouths.

The story was dreadful; it was too horrible to listen further. I was repelled by the whole situation. In fact, I found myself wondering if some of this were fabricated, even though I knew that these specific details had been corroborated. When I am confronted with stories as hard to hear as this, one of my responses can be to close down and distance myself from what I have heard. I understand this withdrawal to be both a form of self-protection and a primitive denial that anything quite this revolting could ever happen. But, when I pay attention to what has been recounted, I know without doubt that evil has been perpetrated on these children. Are the children innocent in this situation? Of course they are. They had no control over how they were treated; they depended entirely on the adults around them to keep them safe. Not surprisingly, this very young boy has already been noted to be aggressive toward his peers and has been identified as having a "behavior problem"; he is labeled as a "bad boy." What is his future? Can he recover? Is healing possible?

My experience with my adolescent patients has taught me that many juvenile offenders report similar childhood stories of abuse and neglect. It is all too common a situation. Seen this way, the enormity of it becomes appalling. These two little children have a strong likelihood of growing up to be themselves perpetrators of evil. My troubled adolescent patients carry the burden of the evil done to them earlier in their lives; they both carry the burden and pass it on. I have no way to deal with these devastating patterns of antisocial behavior except under the label of evil, which I understand to be the complete absence of God and God's goodness. At the same time, my faith compels me to believe that good (that is, God) can overcome evil, though I certainly do not know how or when this might be. The interventions I have learned to use have to do with healing and alleviating suffering. I do what I know how to do, and I learn on the job again and again the multiple ways that God may act, my learning limited only by my ability to perceive and to comprehend. It is patients like Ann and families like Mandy's who show me God's presence in the midst of their suffering.

When I consider what it is that compels me to believe in God, I am aware of an urgency behind my faith which does not seem to come from me. I recognize the force of the drive to believe as coming from somewhere other than myself; I cannot define it further except to know it is God's will for me. My sureness of

God and God's goodness may seem at times to be simple optimism, but it is much more than that. It is grounded in faith supported by liturgy and by corporate worship. It is constantly renewed by God's world around me: the sheer natural beauty of the world, the constancy of the universe through the centuries, the predictability of the seasons, the unvarying cycle of nights and days. I am sustained by the human capacity for creative beauty in all the arts. I am strengthened by my family and our love for each other. And, not least, my interactions with my patients provide me with a very special sense of God's love, which in large part is what keeps me coming to work each day.

Families come to our clinics from the immediate community and also from a wide area of rural Virginia. Sometimes these are people I know well from previous visits; sometimes we have never met before. Often the given reason for the visit is relatively simple. The medical encounter goes well; then, not infrequently, comes the "Oh, by the way" question, after the family and I have established some mutual respect and trust. Now I may hear their more intimate concerns and fears. I remember a little boy I shall call Kenny, who lived in the country about an hour's drive away. He was brought in by his mother because the school had been complaining about his behavior and had raised the question of whether he needed treatment with Ritalin for an attention deficit disorder. Kenny's mother was straightforward and seemed competent. After exploring Kenny's health and developmental history, I asked her about the family situation. She told me they were staying with relatives while their new home was being built. Her boyfriend, who is not Kenny's father, was staying there too. She acknowledged that this living situation was stressful. Kenny was by far the youngest in the household, and everyone had expectations of him, if indeed they noticed him at all. When I asked directly about violence, she admitted that her boyfriend had hit Kenny. "But he was drunk," she quickly added, as if that excused it. Clearly this was a complex situation, which medications were not going to cure. It was also possible that some of Kenny's difficulties would resolve when they moved into the new house, but the boyfriend's drinking and violence would still be there. We discussed some simple parenting issues for her to work on and I asked her to return for follow-up.

At the next visit, Kenny's mother was very upset and obviously close to tears. I talked with Kenny briefly to hear any concerns of his, and then asked him to spend some time with our clinic teacher in the waiting room while his mother and I did some "grown-up" talking. She then told me that Kenny's behavior had become much worse. He had been suspended from school after being violent in the classroom. Her boyfriend had been charged with driving under the influence of alcohol and had lost his license. He had moved away and their relationship had crumbled. The new house was an impossible dream. She stopped talking and started to cry. I found my box of tissues. I touched her gently on the arm to let her know I was still there, still with her. Gradually, the tears subsided and I could feel a bond between us as we connected very quietly. She had shared with me her pain and I could hold it with her. She was not alone; I was aware that God was with us and carrying this burden, too. I helped her identify some immediate resources so that she could move forward beyond this point.

The feeling of being connected to my patients in this quiet way occurs from time to time, and it is a very special and rewarding experience for me. On reflection, I realize that I may even deliberately work toward achieving such a connection for its therapeutic value to the family as well as to me. A common situation comes to mind, when I can almost predict that a connection will occur. I am frequently consulted about the possibility of sexual abuse of young children who spend time in different households because their parents have separated. There is often distinct antagonism between the families. The child, typically a preschooler, may have complained of having a sore bottom. Could this be from molestation? Even before I examine the child, I know that I am unlikely to find definitive signs of abuse; such findings are rare. Most often the examination is normal or shows at most some nonspecific genital irritation, a finding most likely to have been caused by inadequate hygiene and relatively common in little girls for whom there are no suspicions of abuse. However, in a given situation, I cannot prove any of this one way or the other from my examination. Without a clear answer, the family is left to worry about one of the most emotionally difficult issues in child rearing. I cannot tell them whether or not their child has been molested, but I can share with them the horrible difficulty of having to let one's child be in a situation outside one's control, particularly when there is no trust or respect between the families. If I can find the right words, if the family has been able to move with me through the process inherent in the visit, there may be a moment of connection between us, a sudden mutual recognition of sharing that may allow each of us to move on.

I have recounted the last two stories to illustrate how I am both sustained and renewed by my work with my patients. These moments of connection are extremely gratifying and precious to me. When I reflect more on what is happening, I recognize that the connections come at times of intense emotional sharing. They may arise from some immense sadness, as in the first of these two stories, or from some profound anxiety, some fearful loss of control, as in the second. The connection may also come at a time of great joy. For one month each year, I am the attending doctor in our newborn nursery. When everything has gone well or when, despite some real difficulties, the baby is fine, the sense of relief and joy is immense. Some families spontaneously give thanks to God. Others, after some small gesture of sharing from me, quietly agree that this is a miracle, God-given. This is one of the very few occasions when I may speak to a family of my own sense of "God with us," as we make a connection based on joy in the baby's birth.

I have come to recognize that God is present to me at these times of connection, and perhaps also present to the family. I recognize these times as "moments of grace," given by God. I savor them. I am increasingly aware that my faith in God is the basis of my life, albeit at a particularly private level of my being. It is not something I talk about easily, yet I can readily acknowledge the presence of God in my work. God is always there, even though I am not always ready to know God. My patients may tell me how God acts in their lives. I myself perceive God's presence at the times of connection I call moments of grace. There have been times of great stress in my life when it was hard to hear more stories of suffering, to carry more burdens. My own woes competed for my attention and even threatened to overwhelm me. I found God absent, not there to buoy me up. At those times, I could not do my work; I could not bear the burdens alone. I had first to find healing for myself, to reconnect with God before I could presume once again to offer care to others.

My life is rich and I am blessed; I know God's goodness. At the same time, I cannot avoid coming up against evil. I can shun it, but it is nevertheless all around us at every level of existence. Day by day, I am presented with unavoidable evidence of evil in the sufferings of my patients. If I choose to ignore the evil, I may protect myself from the horror of the story, but that does not diminish its impact on my patients; the evil is still there. I must choose to acknowledge the evil and even to confront it directly if I am to provide the care sought from me as a doctor, to share the suffering and to ease the burden of my patients' pain. I can do this day after day only with God's help, by being open to knowing God's will from my patients and through my connections to them, open to receiving the precious moments of grace.

Thus, I know how God is present to me in my work. I know that I can bear to hear my patients' suffering, to share their heavy burdens and search for ways to help them cope, only if I myself am strong. The strength is from God.

3

The Tragedy of "Why Me, Doctor?"

Julia E. Connelly

In this chapter I shall explore two related issues: first, *tragedy*, with attention to the definition and the application of the term in various situations, and second, the question "*Why me?*" as we consider why bad things happen. This exploration will be done against the clinical backdrop of the primary care of adult patients, the field known as general internal medicine. This area of medicine cares for a spectrum of persons, from those who are healthy to those dying of chronic disabling diseases. I have been a general internist for twenty years and have practiced in a rural community for fifteen years. I shall consider tragedy in relation to patients, their families, and the community through my experience as a primary care physician. I shall then look at clinical issues related to the question "Why me?" asked by patients, and associated questions asked by family members trying to understand why bad things happen to those they love.

To begin the discussion of tragedy, I suggest that two sources of information will be necessary for us to proceed. First, as onlookers to a specific situation, we need access to the story, the central feature of this discussion. Through the story we obtain a description of the situation: What happened? What is the plot or theme? Who are the featured characters? How and why are they involved? What are their decisions and choices, and what are the consequences of these decisions and choices? What is the motivation for their involvement or role in the story? When and where does the story take place? Who tells the story? How universal are the basic issues experienced in the story: the conflicts, the losses, the suffering, the horror? Second, Bouchard[1] describes some of the elements of tragedy that may be contained within a story that is told or an event that is observed. Although he writes that "tragedy resists definition," he describes three elements of tragedy explored in Greek plays: (1) the suffering of the individual or individuals involved, (2) the choices made leading toward the tragic outcome, and (3) the aspects of a situation that are beyond the limits of our understanding, e.g., concerns about "Why me?" or "How can this be?" As the story evolves, specific features of the story need to be accessible, such as those unexpected, unpredictable, incomprehensible occurrences that often involve unfortunate choices and lead to suffering.

Another aspect of tragedy, as of many other sorts of stories, is its tendency to elicit emotional reactions that have universal characteristics. These reactions are experienced by those directly involved—the main characters or, as in a theatrical performance, the main actors. They are also experienced by observers, as in the case of an audience watching the performance of a tragic Greek drama, or by family members, friends, and the community of onlookers who witness the story. Characteristic emotional responses include intense identification with the main characters of the story through feelings of love, compassion, pain, and suffering. Often there is a longing to reach out, to help, or even a wish to trade places. The sympathetic and empathic reactions toward the characters are often in themselves dramatic. The horror that arises from the situation and that accompanies the realization of the universal possibility of the event—it could happen to anyone—is an unmistakable response. There are feelings of hopelessness or powerlessness and often angry outbursts against God from whom only *good* things are expected by some. Individuals' values, expectations, and assumptions about the world, their spiritual connections, and religious beliefs are often turned upside down by the tragic events. These reactions embody the universal quality and commonality of the experience of tragedy.

Tragedy in General Internal Medicine

The first time I remember considering tragedy in medicine was during my later years of medical education, during my residency. Now I can recall numerous tragedies that occurred while I was in medical school, but at the time I did not recognize or categorize the situations as tragedies. The infant whom we diagnosed with leukemia during my third year of medical school, for instance: I grieved for that child so much that I excluded pediatrics from my list of possible career choices. "How could anyone take care of dying children?" I wondered. I felt the emotions of that tragic situation—the sadness, anger, hopelessness, powerlessness, the incomprehensibility of it all. Now, twenty-five years later, I understand that a child's dying of leukemia before learning to walk is a tragedy. But, at the time no one used the word *tragedy*, so I did not label the child's diagnosis and death as such.

Following completion of my residency, I worked as an emergency room physician. Early one cold, rainy evening a call notified us that there had been a head-on collision nearby. Three people involved in the accident were coming in by rescue squad. The nurses and I readied the trauma room and braced ourselves for the unknown. The automatic doors of the ambulance entrance opened; rescue squad attendants rushed in and on to the trauma room. Standing at the head of the stretcher, I looked down on a teenager, a young woman. She did not move, and her pale, bluish face was expressionless. She was not breathing and she had no pulses. I pressed my hands beneath her head preparing to intubate her. As my hands moved forward, her neck felt as if there were no vertebrae, just muscles ineffectively attempting to stabilize her head. My heart sank, and a heavy awareness engulfed me. "Next," I said, realizing that she was dead and that we needed to see if there was someone we could help. Next was an elderly man, also the dreaded DOA—dead on arrival. The third one I never saw; he was "fine."

There was little for us to do. Our jobs were over quickly. We moved about in a stunned silence. A little while later, the door opened again, unexpectedly this time. The young woman's mother entered. She was distraught, needing comfort and understanding. The nurses asked her to come into my office, where we sat with her quietly as she cried. I wondered what in the world I could say that would help or even be appropriate. Soon she asked me, "Why?" She explained that her daughter was a high school student and had been at home all day working on a term paper. She was a good student and worked very hard. In the evening when she was finished writing, she asked if she could go out with her boyfriend. Her mother didn't want her to because it was then dark and rainy, but her daughter had worked hard all day, so she had given her permission. Now she regretted that decision, more than any other in her entire life. "Why?" she asked desperately again.

Now it was my turn to say something to her. The notion of tragedy rose in my mind, the letters flashing before me as I remembered an earlier experience. So I said, "Your daughter's death is a tragedy," acknowledging the horror that we felt and the incomprehensibility of the situation. We listened as she told us about her daughter. There were few words that I could offer, but the idea of tragedy, interwoven with the ideas of loss, suffering, choices, and the limits of our ability to understand, seemed to bring all of us some comfort. She continued to ask "Why?" but she never pushed me for the nonexistent answers. Later one of the nurses thanked me. She said that she had never heard "tragedy" used in the emergency room, but she thought it described the situation well.

Several years earlier, during my residency, I had learned about tragedy, a lesson that helped me that evening in the emergency room. I worked with a cardiologist. One day he asked me to see several patients in consultation, gathering the clinical information and the lab data, while he performed a routine catheterization. We decided to meet about three o'clock that afternoon to make patient rounds, but at three o'clock he was not there. I waited, wondering if something was wrong. After a while he arrived, looking pale, stressed, and hurried. We sat down together in a private conference room, and he explained to me that complications had developed during the catheterization; the patient had died. The family members were on their way to the conference room.

The patient was a very vigorous seventy-six-year-old man, married, retired from a successful family business. He and his wife loved to travel and visit with their children and grandchildren. The previous day he was admitted to the hospital because of a brief episode of atypical chest pain. There had been no cardiac damage, but the decision was made to reevaluate his coronary arteries. The patient and his family agreed and everyone thought that he would be fine, that the pain was probably of a noncardiac origin.

When the family arrived to discuss what had happened during the procedure, my colleague, the cardiologist, expressed his sorrow and told the family once again of the patient's death. He described the details of the procedure and answered their questions. Finally, he described the event and their loss as a tragedy. No one expected this to happen; there was no way to predict it. The man's death was not explainable. The family members asked some more questions, and we said goodbye to them feeling miserable, too. The idea of tragedy stayed with me, and so did many thoughts and feelings related to this patient.

Recognizing Tragedy

Some situations will be described as tragedies by most people. I expect that no matter how we specifically define tragedy, most will agree that the term fits the case of the hardworking high school student who died in the automobile accident on that rainy evening. The accident was unexpected, unpredictable—although her mother was concerned about the weather conditions—and undeserved in one so young and innocent. Most who hear this story will respond to the horror of the experience. A universal reaction of sorrow is felt. Then, from the recognition that this could have happened to me or my child, a panic arises from the realization of this universal possibility. The horror and fear touch almost everyone. Yet, the accident was in many ways a common event, an automobile collision occurring within a few miles of home.

There are others who suffered in this story, too. Perhaps their stories also represent tragedies: How can we know? To continue reflection on the notion of tragedy, consider a few possibilities. What about the young woman's mother and the decision to let her daughter go out that rainy evening? Her decision was, I suggest, a personal tragedy for her. Her daughter is dead now and she feels the responsibility, loss, and blame for the situation. There is little doubt that she regretted her decision and wished that she had said no to her daughter's request. There are other losses in the story, about which we can speculate. What of the young woman's boyfriend, the driver of the car? Was this also a tragedy for him, since he was confronted with the death of a friend and perhaps with legal consequences as well? And what of the elderly man who was also DOA? Was his death a tragedy, too? Here we see numerous stories unfolding. There are stories about the accident and those involved, then the beginning of the stories that help the survivors process the situation. For instance, the young woman's mother may begin to reconstruct the events, wishing that she had made a different decision.

The discussion, I think, gets much more difficult as we struggle to define tragedy. How can we know what constitutes a tragedy, when we know so little about the person? The young woman's death is a tragedy; we know enough of her situation in life to realize the loss and unfulfilled dreams. But the elderly man comes to us with no information of his life, his longings, his dreams. The outcome—his death—does not by itself constitute a tragedy. Death can be a natural and welcomed event. What if he had actually had a heart attack and died just prior to the impact of the accident—a natural death, in other words? Then we might note his age and his luck in dying quickly without suffering. But what if he were traveling to his only daughter's wedding the following day? Or to his great-grandson's birth? What then of tragedy, of age and dreams? And what is the response of his family when they hear of the accident and his death?

A closer look at the case of the man who died during the cardiac catheterization might reveal that the physician described the situation as a tragedy as much for himself as for the patient's family. After all, he recommended the procedure. It was his choice to try to eliminate uncertainty for the patient, to define the origin of his chest pain. Although the patient agreed to the procedure and probably understood the potential risks, the physician made the initial recommendation to proceed. Without knowing the patient it is hard to define his death as a tragedy, although it may have been. Despite his age, he was actively engaged in living. Children, grandchildren, hobbies, travels, dreams: perhaps the fact that his life ended abruptly while he was still so involved makes his death a tragedy. But we really know very little about the meaning of his life, or about his daily existence at that time.

These cases present dramatic events in the lives of the patients and their families and their physicians. Tragedies are often dramatic events that involve unexpected, unpredictable occurrences and choices that result in suffering. There are many examples of tragedies that fit this description—airline crashes, bombings, murders of innocent bystanders. Would anyone argue about the tragic nature of these situations and the individual tragedies experienced in these events? These situations push us to the limits of our ability to understand why bad things happen. Individual or personal choices—e.g., decisions about when, where, and how to travel—must be confronted by family members and friends. The concern about individual suffering of the victims is a source of stress for survivors. Surviving families, friends, and communities suffer, too.

Such tragedies influence the health of a community and its members. In our community recently a woman was kidnapped from a busy highway where she had apparently been lured into thinking that her car was malfunctioning. After much community effort to find her, including television reports, newspaper stories, wanted posters of the suspect, and dog searches, her body was found buried in a shallow grave. Not too long after her abduction and death, two young women were found dead, murdered on the Appalachian Trail in an adjacent county. Two other murders, both of elderly women, occurred in the nearby area. The community as a whole was disturbed by these murders. All of these situations could be described as tragedies, and the tragedies had many characters: the victims, their families and friends, and the community. How could these things happen in our community? How could people be so cruel as to murder or abduct innocent people? The community members suffered. In the office I saw a number of patients who suffered along with the victims and their families. Some developed feelings of hopelessness and depression. Several older women expressed fear of living in their homes alone, discussing issues of safety and feelings of vulnerability. One patient was unable to drive alone, and decided to fly rather than drive on a trip to avoid the risk of being kidnapped from her car. People spoke with a lot of anxiety and sadness about the situation in general.

The performance of Greek tragedies arouses emotional responses such as anger, fear, and distrust among audience participants. Themes of powerlessness, disappointment, despair, and grief offer common grounds for communal identification with the ones who suffer. In the recent tragedies I've described, as in Greek tragedies, the community as a whole responded to and identified with the universal nature of the suffering and the potential for such events to happen to anyone in the community.

These dramatic situations are tragedies. But many clinical situations that result in pain, suffering, and loss may not be so easily recognized as tragedies; they may be so embedded in our everyday lives that they are not identified as such. The idea of "everyday tragedies" offers one explanation of my former perception that few tragedies occur in primary care medicine. Medical ethics has struggled with a similar dichotomy: dramatic tertiary care ethics cases versus primary care cases.[2] Dramatic cases, usually situated in tertiary care hospitals, of anencephalic infants or of brain-dead persons on life support are well known, while cases from primary care have been described as "everyday," as if they are not of critical importance. Everyday ethical issues and everyday tragedies are embedded in the everyday life of the community. The ethical issues may be inseparable from personal and cultural beliefs and values commonly held by the community, while everyday tragedies may be a part of usual life—illness, accidents, and "bad" things happening to individuals and families. For instance, I recently had a long discussion with a woman whose daughter had gotten married without informing her. This withholding by the daughter, the separation and demonstration of the distance in their relationship, was unexpected, unpredicted, and unexplainable by the mother. She was devastated by it, but held in her feelings for six months until she felt compelled to tell her daughter how she felt. The confrontation entailed the risk of losing her daughter, but she realized that had already happened. Other examples include the person unable to afford medication needed to prevent asthma exacerbations and pregnant women who do not receive prenatal care. We are surrounded by episodes of abuse—physical, sexual, verbal, and other. Neglect of the elderly is a tragedy. Children living with alcoholic or unsupportive or unloving parents live out tragedies. All these unfortunately rather common experiences are tragedies. These everyday issues are broader, grayer, less dramatic, and more a part of the everyday routine than those nationally recognized tragedies or examples from tertiary care hospitals. But these more subtle issues are also more integral to the world and life of the patient. In this characterization of ethics and tragedy as everyday, we must be cautious not to imply the "ho-hum" quality of a routine or repeated event. Without careful reflection we may ignore or neglect situations in which our ethical concern should be triggered or, in the case of tragedy, we may not feel for the other person as we should. There are many examples of such situations but, until writing this chapter, I had not conceptualized these issues, experiences, and events as tragedies; now I think they are.

Why Me, Doctor?

One aspect of tragedy, addressed in the question "Why me?" is the need to comprehend, to order, and to bring some control to the situation. Implied in the world of the one who asks the question "Why me?" is a belief of some type, probably religious, that bad things should not happen, that God or some higher being should be taking better care of me.

During the fifteen years that I have practiced general internal medicine in a rural community, only a few patients or the events surrounding them stand out as tragedies. And very few patients have asked me to explain why this has happened to them: "Why me?" Using the concept that tragedies are unexpected, unpredictable, undeserved, and unexplainable events that usually involve intense suffering, the fact that I can recall few tragedies or few instances in which patients ask "Why me?" seems odd. This fact is even more striking when you consider the prevalence of suffering, loss, disappointment, and pain in primary care practice.

In order to understand this observation, I began to consider possible explanations. In general, what factors may influence patients to ask this question or not? I assume that the relationship between the patient and the physician is one important variable. If the patient feels safe, confident that the physician will listen to anything that is asked or expressed as a concern, then the patient, it seems to me, will be more likely to ask. The length of the relationship and the depth of previous discussions set the stage for a discussion of "Why me?" but may not be an essential or limiting feature if safety and compassion are felt by the patient. I wonder if this question is asked more commonly in one area of medicine than another. Is it more common in pediatrics, for example, or in the case of cancer patients? Is there something about the nature of general internal medicine that makes discussions of tragedy less likely? Or am I doing something that limits such discussions? Should I be looking for or encouraging this question when patients are diagnosed with chronic or fatal diseases?

In general internal medicine practice there are a number of reasons that this question may not be asked too commonly. Patients using internal medicine practices experience many expected and predictable events, most of which are chronic, occurring over years. With this perspective, patients make adjustments slowly and steadily to their declining health. Many chronic illnesses occur from poor health habits, such as alcohol or tobacco abuse and sedentary lifestyles. So, for many internal medicine patients diseases are predictable, perhaps not tragic, except with respect to persons' inability to change or to take care of themselves for whatever reason. Also, many general medicine patients are elderly and, although disease is a burden at any age, the development of breast cancer at 80 is usually perceived to be less of a tragedy than when the diagnosis is made in a young person. But there are also chronic diseases that occur unexpectedly and without any particular reason; for instance, patients with rheumatoid arthritis may suffer greatly as the illness progresses. Although I follow a large number of patients with chronic degenerative conditions, many were diagnosed prior to my involvement with them, so discussions about "Why me?" may have taken place with an earlier physician.

Reynolds Price, an acclaimed American novelist, poet, and playwright, published in 1994 *A Whole New Life*, an account of his struggle to survive a spinal cord tumor. He discusses the question "Why me?" and provides another perspective on the perceived absence of such a question in my practice. He writes:

> But with all the morbidity of such parlor games, some vital impulse spared my needing to reiterate the world's most frequent and pointless question in the face of disaster—*Why? Why me?* I never asked it; the only answer is of course *Why not?* And a lifetime's exposure to the rocky luck of my large family had inoculated me against the need to make an equally frequent claim—that my fate was unfair or unjust. Aware of the troubles of so many likable kinsmen around me in childhood and youth, I'd almost never expected fairness.[3]

Learning from Patients

Just as I began my reflection on the issue for this chapter, a patient asked, "Why me, Dr. Connelly? Why me?" I'll tell her story as she told it to me that day and follow it along for a few weeks as a way to make several observations about important points that I learned from her.

When I first met her, she was sixty-five years old and recently diagnosed with presumed lung cancer. The previous year a mass had been noted on a CT scan of her chest while she was in the hospital, but she refused further diagnostic evaluation. After her discharge she was referred to me. Each time she came in we talked about the mass, discussed its likely cause, and reviewed the steps needed to make a definite diagnosis. She understood all of this, including the information that the likely diagnosis was lung cancer and that it was incurable in its present state, but that some palliative interventions might slow its progress. However, each time we spoke she refused evaluation because she was feeling fine, despite having back pain, which she blamed on a procedure performed during her initial hospital stay.

Finally, the day came when she no longer felt well, and she agreed to have a biopsy. That day in the office she asked me, "Why me, Dr. Connelly? Why me?" I knew it was an important question for her, so I reflected it back to her. This is the story of our discussion. I did not have a tape recorder; it is reported as I recall it.

Patient: I had a fall and hurt my back.

Doctor: So you think that has something to do with the tumor?

P: It could. The devil was there.

D: How do you mean, the devil?

P: You see, I had this tree. I knew I shouldn't climb it, being sixty-five and all. But I saw the ladder and went up anyway and cut the limb. The devil enticed me into that tree and then I fell and hurt my back.

D: So you are blaming yourself for following the devil, falling, and developing cancer from the injury?

P: Yes, I guess so.

D: I don't know; maybe it just happened or it was just bad luck.

P: So what is the mass?

D: I can't really say without a biopsy, but I'm sure it is lung cancer of some type.

P: I've been really scared of having lung cancer. My father had lung cancer and so did others in the family. I remember watching him die. I quit smoking thirty years ago; I didn't want cancer.

I was surprised by her story. First, she blamed herself for having this tumor because she had followed the devil: If only she had not climbed the tree and fallen, she would not have received an injury that she believed resulted in the cancer's activation. As we talked on, she expressed her belief that her faith had not been strong enough, and she was to blame for the fall. Second, she understood that her smoking could have caused the cancer. Yet, she had done what she could at the time to prevent cancer; she had stopped smoking thirty years ago. Now she needed to reconcile her understanding of God as she questioned, "How can God do this to me?"

She agreed to have a biopsy and she was diagnosed with lung cancer. Radiation was recommended and, after much consideration, she decided to undergo this treatment. Several weeks later she returned to the office. As we talked I asked her how she was doing with the question of "Why me?" "Oh, that question," she said, appearing ashamed. "I don't know how I could have been so bold to question God. I can't believe I even asked. You know that I'm going to radiation every day. Well, there are many of us older folks who go like me, but there is one young boy, nine years old. When I saw him the first time I began to thank God for my sixty-eight years; I'll never ask why again."

I learned many lessons from her. She asked "Why me?" at a time when I had a heightened interest, so when she returned I chose to inquire about our initial conversation and asked for her further reflections. Now I understand her perspective and her thankfulness regarding her long life. She has completed or at least expanded her understanding of her story. This working through, this retelling is another important function of stories for the individual, as it moves them into a process of healing, in her case spiritual healing. The impact of her work and disclosure of these stories on my relationship with her has been surprising to me. Knowing her story and understanding her resolution have been very helpful to me in caring for her. I feel very peaceful with her, as I know that she is at peace with her illness.

I now suspect that many, perhaps most, people at least think about asking "Why me?" when bad things like illnesses and accidents occur, but many personal and interpersonal factors influence its expression. The question does seem to require a belief system that says "Bad things will not happen to me, if . . ."

Conclusion

The concept of tragedy is important to integrate into the physician's professional world. Since many events are not explainable, the notion of tragedy allows the physician to remain open to the possibility of not knowing or not having answers in such situations. No one is responsible for having an explanation of why "bad" or tragic events occur. With this open attitude, the emotions of the situation can be experienced and shared by both patient and physician; comfort and support can be expressed. Movement toward surviving and healing, rather than explaining, can begin.

My patient with lung cancer died recently after her long illness. She remained thankful for the years she had lived, rather than angry or hopeless about her "doomed" future. I understood her peaceful state of being, because I had had the opportunity to explore with her the question "Why me?" With the presentation of bad news, such as a diagnosis of lung cancer, physicians observe many reactions in their patients. Some individuals feel hopeless and depressed, others become very anxious and fearful, while others experience the peacefulness associated with certainty. Often it is difficult to understand a person's response: Is her quiet acceptance a flight into health? Is the anxiety due to his fear of what is to come, the unknowable next moment?

My experience with this patient resulted in a clearer understanding of her because I knew her story and shared in her awareness. This process changed my role in her life and further medical care. Our visits were more personal and more focused on the truth of the experience for her than is the case in many patients' visits. I became more certain about ways to help her as her illness progressed. When "bad" news is shared or tragedy occurs, perhaps the physician could inquire at the appropriate time, "Have you ever asked yourself 'Why me?'" Many patients may not ask, possibly afraid of the inevitable response: "Why not!" But, for those who have begun the questioning, asking them about it may open the door for a conversation that will facilitate understanding.

How can physicians learn to encourage patients to share these intimate stories? Using literature in medical education helps students explore the world of the patient[4]—the wide range of experiences and reactions that individuals have in association with events in their lives, illnesses, and accidents. Gregory Orr, a poet and professor of English at the University of Virginia, writes about the role of disorder in our lives: "Poetry and especially lyric poetry is a 'translation' of the interplay of order and disorder out of life and into language."[5] Tragedy is certainly one example of disorder as it occurs randomly and without reason. Yet, all of us need order; our minds respond to disorder with attempts to reorder, as in the question "Why me?" Here we look for the order, the reason for the event. Orr argues that the poet must allow the disorder in. As a physician, I suggest that patients and physicians must let the disorder of the experience into their beings to feel and experience its turmoil. Admitting disorder allows other inquiries to happen: The patient with lung cancer, in the midst of her questioning and despair, experienced the joy of having lived a rather long life. Orr claims that the poet survives because the disorder is admitted into the poet's life and experience, and I add that the patient (and perhaps the physician) can survive and heal by inquiry into the question "Why me?" as they define and develop the whole story.[6]

4

When Truth Is Mediated by a Life

Albert H. Keller

In places where pastors and health professionals are busy attending the needs of sick, dying, or bereaved people, the theological conundrum of how one can assert both the goodness and the omnipotence of God in the face of suffering is a background issue. A clinical chaplain emphasized the foreground issue when we were talking recently about a patient. "They want a companion in crisis, not a chaplain to give an answer," he said. "Nancy asked all the questions—Why does God allow this to happen to me?—and I attempted to answer them, but she didn't want that. She wanted someone to validate the questions." He added that sometimes it is also his role to help the patient ask those hard questions, by not discounting their ventures onto hazardous ground and by encouraging and lending language to express their anguish or their anger. In this way, he said, we respect the person's integrity in her unique relationship to God.

The chaplain was focused on the person. He interpreted her questions as expressions of existential needs and sized his responses to fit what he believed was troubling her soul. We may agree that Nancy's question, at the moment of her asking, is more like a cry than a query. And yet the ineluctable question remains—Why does God allow this to happen to me? That is the question that must be validated by the chaplain. Background or foreground, the theodicy question impinges on the mind in times of suffering. It is not the intellectual history of the question that impinges, but its immediate power to shape the sufferer's experience of the divine in her life and to frame her capacity to meet the present crisis. That is the reason I approach theodicy as a faith question, not as a philosophical conundrum. In a clinical setting, where such questions come embodied in personal narratives, the struggle to understand the nature and ways of God amid suffering and sorrow is absolutely pertinent to the lived integrity of both patient and clinician.

Living as we do under conditions by which we see in a glass darkly and not face to face, our conceptions of God are analogical. What analogs or metaphors, then, are most truthful in speaking of God in relation to our perceptions of evil in the world? What language shall we borrow to make sense out of our most conflicting human experience?

That question will guide my retelling of a conversation I had with Drew, a man whose personal narrative provides both cause to ask the theodicy question and rich metaphors for a response to it. Drew's only biological child was born ten years ago with significant birth defects. Today the child is mentally and physically handicapped; he is also loved and cared for at home as an integral part of the family. The family includes a healthy younger daughter, a child whose birth history had put her at significant risk of handicap and whom the couple adopted with that possibility in view.

Drew is not only the father of a severely handicapped child. He is also a scientist, a nuclear fusion physicist who practices at the interface of theoretical physics and the practicalities of corporate business. The link between the two domains, according to Drew, is nonlinear dynamics, and the mediator is the digital computer. One senses the presence of the computer in his conversation as one would likely sense the presence of the violin in conversation with Isaac Stern. Note Drew's immersion in the two domains of science and business. Science and business define the two dominant mentalities of contemporary Western culture. Attending to this conversation with Drew, we overhear the voice of a society that is saturated with scientific rationality and marketplace practicality—but that is also still open, perhaps increasingly so, to God. Men and women whose practices exemplify the dominant spirit of the time, yet who are also persons of faith seeking understanding, can give crucial theological signals at a time when traditional authorities are no longer taken as compelling. That is, such women and men indicate to us how great questions can be answered, and truth mediated, not in dogma, but in a life.

Conversation is the native soil of the clinical enterprise. Clinicians are accustomed to joining their personally grounded and disciplined perspectives with the responses of the patient, client, or parishioner in an effort to achieve what Spence calls "narrative truth."[1] This aspect of clinical method, undergirded by the assumption that truth can indeed be mediated by a life, controls this investigation into the problem of suffering.

The following account comprises three conversations between Drew and myself; his wife was occasionally present. The conversations took place in Drew's home over successive weeks, approximately three hours in all, audiotaped and transcribed. I then drew the conversations together into a narrative summary. Drew and his wife read the summary with a view to amending the narrative to express Drew's thought more accurately. The amended version has been abridged, with names and identifying details altered, but not substantively changed in the account that follows. The conscious theme of our conversation was not theodicy; we were discussing the intersections of science and religious faith in Drew's biographical experience. In the clinical and pastoral arenas, it often happens that way: We learn about God and evil obliquely, when we thought we were talking about something else.

The Conversations

Drew works in an analysis group at the laboratory of a communications company. He describes his workplace as a "data warehouse for all different kinds of core pieces of information that the company needs to run the business." The data range from marketing and service orders to the full appraisal of the traffic on the communications network: "Just a tremendous amount of information—trying to bring all this stuff together." Drew is currently attempting to build an integrated view of customer activity based on the types of service the company provides. His work is meaningful to him in ways that justify calling it a "practice," as Alasdair MacIntyre uses the term.[2]

Having heard Drew's description of his work, I wondered to what degree the data analysis he was doing in the marketplace calls upon his training and research in physics. The bridge between the two domains, he explained, is a methodological one. Problems in physics seem *cleaner* than problems in the marketplace, where they are more "highly dimensional." Marketplace problems demand more "robust" techniques for analysis, meaning techniques that are less sensitive to errors in determining underlying distribution patterns, that is, in "pulling information out of the noise." Pressed for an example, Drew displayed his theoretical base:

> In physics, you could be trying to model a shock wave propagating through some deforming material. There are a lot of complex issues, but you can sit down and put the various important pieces together that you have to model, . . . using your static grid to model the information, or some grid that moves with the shock wave. It's a lot of high-level engineering calculus, but it's do-able. Now you get over into marketing issues, you don't know what to do! You have all the, say, stock prices, one marketing issue; you can have all the fundamental drivers that drive prices, in terms of tax laws and business cycles and the relative strength of competition—all those fundamental drivers—but then you have all the nonlinear feedback of people's fears and greeds, and perception being nine tenths of reality, all of that stuff. *It's a very chaotic system.* It has its external drivers but it also has all this nonlinear feedback. So marketing issues would be a lot more chaotic than physical science issues.

I noted that Drew characterized the market as a "chaotic system." He was careful not to allow me to stamp his thoughts with the label "chaos theory." Knowing I was a layman, he feared the popular term would "overload the word with people's traditional [common] meaning, where they have a close association of chaos and randomness." Markets are not random, he insisted; there is value derived from analyzing the data. More correctly, chaos is "a driven system with nonlinear feedback" in which one cannot account for all the processes individually that contribute to the product. Using the example of the turbulent motion of fluid in a pipe, he explained:

> If you sat down and looked at the characteristic sizes of any set form, the swirls would disappear. . . . Looking at the inertia of the fluid, viscosity, the flow velocity, the diameter of the pipe . . . one person might say, "What causes this result, the inertia or the viscosity?" The question doesn't make any sense. It's a dynamic system. It's not just one component that's responsible for effects.

Drew expanded his description of the market as a chaotic system by alluding to what has become known as the "butterfly effect."

> People have the view that big events have big consequences and insignificant events have insignificant consequences. But you get to chaos theory, and you see *the infinite sensitivity of the future to the present.* You begin to appreciate the fact that there's no threshold of consequences to events, in terms of no limit to the influence they can have.

One of the interesting features of Drew's conversation was the fluidity in his transitions from physical principles, particularly the chaos principle, to business analysis and, more interesting to me, to moral and theological ideas and their social embodiment in his family life. When he spoke of the "infinite sensitivity of the future to the present," he used the illustration of the sneeze today that averts the tornado six months from now, and even the unpredictable but real consequences of greeting someone with "Hi" rather than "Hello"—the butterfly effect. He then took that notion, hatched in physical chaos theory, to the "profound implications to responsibility, and trying to make amends . . . if you realize what the real system is like." Thus he had come to realize how clouded moral responsibility and accountability appear when one recognizes that people act in dynamic, interactive systems with multiple variables that impinge on any given result.

Drew had located morality within a chaotic system of social behavior. Momentarily brought up short by the implications of that move for my teaching discipline, bioethics, my response singled out the feature of "unpredictability" in what I had heard him say. It was not the time for narrowing down, however. He was thinking theologically. "Yeah. It changes the way you look at life, and God's purpose, and where you think the interface is between God's will and your freedom of choice. Just profoundly core issues."

Core issues? I thought how Drew and his wife had received a severely handicapped baby into their family and incorporated him into the weave of their everyday life—and of their everyday faith. Then they intentionally sought out another child with a difficult beginning and a very uncertain future, provided her foster care, and adopted her when permitted to do so. They would not have chosen for their son to be handicapped, yet the experience of accepting and loving him was essentially related to their choice of providing another at-risk baby a home and a life. Struck by this interface of "God's will" and the couple's freedom of choice, I asked Drew to talk more about how his understanding of chaos affects such "profoundly core issues" as these.

He began his answer as a physicist but was not long in drawing out the theological correlation. When you link chaos theory with quantum field theory, he explained, "all the evidence, and it's well documented, points to the fact that *the present is objectively undetermined.*" Indeterminacy, for Drew, is the tenet of scientific faith that "changes the way you look at life," as he had put it earlier. He spelled out this fundamental idea in terms of the Heisenberg uncertainty principle, which led him to the conclusion that the root of reality is a probability function, not particles or waves or anything other than *the probability of an interaction.* "Which means," he fairly shouted, "there is no such thing as destiny! It's a myth—just an old concept of thinking, that the future can be known. But all of science and technology now point to the fact that the future is open and undetermined, as our intuition tells us it is."

That conclusion is inescapably moral for Drew, who has no difficulty going from "is" to "ought." "It's part of my belief that you're supposed to play the cards you're dealt. I think God's meaning for us is to deal with the universe that we live within, and in that universe there is no such thing as destiny."

Drew's disciplined study of physics pulled him away from the modernist view of a universe governed either by the laws of classical Newtonian mechanics or by a metaphysical determinism identified with God. The chaos principle in combination with quantum physics leads him both intellectually and morally to affirm a world in which creativity is more to the point than control. The human part in the unfolding drama of reality is "to play the cards you're dealt"—which means something totally different from passively accepting one's hand. Interlacing his moral insight and his scientific practice, Drew marveled that human beings are "infinite state machines" in contrast to the finite states, repeatable and predictable, of artificial intelligence. Human thought processes are chaotic in the sense that they are infinitely sensitive to initial conditions (the cards we're dealt), yet even these initial conditions are indeterminate. We are utterly, infinitely open to the world as it is and as it is becoming.

Our action is then truly creative action, free of any pretense of control. "I think one of the real issues of the purpose of life," he said, "is to see that it's not . . . to have a mission of making the world fit your model of what it should look like, because your unintentional, uncontrolled power is significantly greater than your controlled power." Because you cannot control the things of the future, you should direct your energy to "things that you're doing versus what you're trying to control." Since taking a breath can have more impact on the future than amassing a fortune, rein in your ambitions and appreciate reflectively what you are doing now. Drew learned this counsel of mindfulness largely from physics.

Drew's practice of science, and his secondary practice of corporate business, have been the formative matrices of his worldview. Drew is also a person of Christian faith, but he does not hold this faith as something separate from science. Separation of the two domains has been a device for addressing realities that do not seem to fit together. Drew's assumption is different: There is one reality, about which we learn in various ways. His perspective on reality, shaped to a large extent by chaos and quantum field theories, is shaped also by his experience of the divine in his life, including the experience of having been dealt what some observers might call a bad hand. Believing in God was prior to Drew's intellectual grasp of chaos. As his mind was imbued with the perspective of indeterminacy from quantum physics, he became more understanding of a dynamic factor in reality that is creative and calls one to responsibility, something one can trust and worship and follow.

During our discussion of chaos and the nonlinear nature of reality, my thoughts kept returning to a biblical image. I inserted my conjecture into the conversation:

> What it makes me think of is what Jesus said about spirit and the action of the Divine Spirit. "The wind blows where it will and you hear the sound of it, but you know not whence it comes nor whither it goes." The word for spirit in Hebrew is *ruah*, "wind; turbulent flow"! I wonder if the science of turbulent flow is not in some sense an analogy of the way Jesus understood the action of the Holy Spirit?

Drew's response was not personal but cosmological. "Well, the universe runs on chaos. The sun runs on chaos. Our bodies run on chaos." But is the chaos like the action of *ruah*, the Creative Spirit that brooded upon the dark waters, or is it the uncreated and formless void itself? I wanted to know something absolutely fundamental from the faith experience of this reflective scientist. Is there a divine Word—encoded information, unfolding purpose—beyond and within the complexity and chaos of your cosmology?

Drew put that question more bluntly:

> Is God running reality or not? It struck me that it's a core issue. What do I really believe—about misfortune being God's will, or something that God just tolerates, or what? Certainly throughout the Bible you see a lot of people struggling with this issue. You remember the disciple asking Jesus about the man born blind: Was it his sins or was it the sins of his father?

I realized that this question about the causation of a significant birth defect was an existential question for him. I observed simply that the disciple's question appears to have been based on very linear assumptions about causality. Drew then proceeded to comment on the story of the man born blind. In doing so, he disclosed a theodicy similar in at least one aspect to the biblical book of Job: Each ends not in a rational solution to the problem—if we overlook the last chapter of Job—but in an affirmation of beauty.

In the story, Drew recounted, Jesus answered the questioner that the blindness was due to neither postulated cause, but was to show the glory of God. A naive interpretation of that statement would see this unfortunate man's affliction as God's device for teaching other people a lesson. Hard luck for him! Drew dismissed that idea and observed that there are many instances in the Bible, including the story of Job, where an individual's misfortune is thought, at least by some, to have been given to test the sufferer's faith. This way of thinking ascribes a lower level of morality to God than we expect human parents to exercise with their children. We expect parents to protect their children from harm when to do so is within their power. The last phrase may be the key—"within their power." Drew implied a responsibility shared by God and humanity for what reality is. Neither God's will nor human free will can be seen as ultimately responsible for all that is, but each conditions the other. "The closest I can come to an explanation of why bad things sometimes happen is that it's not a joy to God that people suffer, but there are just overriding considerations of free will. You can't have both human free will *and* a fair universe."

Human free will is a concept that corresponds to the indeterminacy of human action—it makes sense in Drew's understanding of reality. But what meaning does "God's will" have in a cosmology of chaos? Drew's response shows a man confessing his inability to see the Creator's "plan," and focusing instead on empirical evidences of "God's love at work" consistent with a dynamic and indeterminate system. His practical reasoning became graceful as he thought the matter through:

> Birth defects, getting stomped on by other people, just from a combination of uncertainty and a bad use of other people's free wills—life is unjust. But I think of First Corinthians: Paul is writing probably about the same topic, saying it's hard for a human being to think you have a complete way of looking at God's plan with all this unjustness and all this unfairness—but dimly, through a mirror, you can see God's love at work. I think Paul had a tremendous amount of inspiration and insight to see that. He's right. There's a whole bunch of wonderful things that are happening, on top of all the unfairness. On top of all the unfairness of life, we're learning how to be compassionate. On top of all our limitations, we're learning how to be cared for. On top of all the uncertainty in life, we are learning to trust, and we're learning responsibility and commitment when other people put their trust in us. We're learning how to forgive. . . . Now, as human beings, the

frustration and the hurt from all our losses prevent us from really getting a clear picture of this. But dimly, through a mirror, I think we can see God's wisdom for making reality be what it is, and as Christians we can begin to understand that God created a universe that's filled with His goodness.

Life is empirically unfair, sometimes harsh in dealing the cards, yet we experience enough goodness and care to point us to God's love at work on a field not yet clearly seen. Drew insisted all along that "chaos" does not mean *random*, but *nonlinear*. That is, amid the complex connections of life that contradict linear notions of just deserts, we get intimations of a higher resolution upon a hidden ground of goodness. Again and again, within that plane of the complex connections of life, Drew the scientist and Drew the theologian pronounced his acceptance of life as he finds it. This is the resolution that reminds me of the book of Job:

> But it's beautiful, you know? I hate death; I hate losing people who die; I hate my own death. Life is so interesting and so much fun, I hate to blow the game. I mean it's one of the true mysteries of life how something that is so unjust and so unfair can be so beautiful. They say truth is beauty; here is injustice as beauty!

To summarize this discussion, the problem Drew calls "free will and God's will" is really the existential question of how we shall live and participate in a world that seems unjust and unfair. There is no malice, he says; both the present and the future are indeterminate. And in accepting both the bad and the good we perceive not omnipotence—monarchical control—but God's creative love in operation all the way through, from the bottom (quantum indeterminacy) to the top (human systems, such as family life). We know this from no external authority but because the conviction rings true—to life, to science, and to spiritual experience.

From the standpoint of the problem of suffering, the second big question that Drew has to deal with is a teleological question. How can we meaningfully speak of purpose within a universe created in self-organizing chaos, in which both present and future are radically open? Is there intentionality in creation? These kinds of questions dominated our third conversation, the most passionate dialogue of all.

Drew is amazed at the fact of life itself—that things evolve, that molecules came together to form organic matter. Short of the existence of life, he is amazed even at a snowflake:

> People don't understand how crystals form. It's not a question of molecules forming geometrical patterns. So you have to be careful in terms of thinking of physical processes as just random occurrences when they have the ability to seek their own goals. The way crystals can build upon themselves, and seek structure—like life, it's goal-seeking.

Most amazing, and most confirming of God's intelligence, is "the incredible balance of how the universe supports life." The basic and necessary ingredient of life is *information*, which requires some basic medium, a coding complex (DNA). How has the universe made within itself a hospitable nest for that fragile possibility? It was when he described the process of stellar evolution that Drew became most animated. "Here's how God did it! Evolution, we'll start with that. Now the physics of a burning star . . ." Drew went on at length, telling the natural history of ten billion years of stellar and then organic evolution. His account held the affection and formality of a liturgy. When I pressed him to say what it is that convinces him of the reality of God in this process, he responded that it is finally the "incredible precision."

> When I look at the universe, I see layer after layer of precision engineering. What does this imply? That we live in a designed universe. There's bull's-eye after bull's-eye after bull's-eye in terms of the whole star evolution process, and we talked before about the precision of the creation of the universe. It's just one incredible feat of precision after another.

Drew never speaks as one who attempts to prove the existence of God by some form of natural theology. He does speak as one who believes in God on other grounds and has been seized by a definite sense of purpose in life. He finds the principle of purposefulness corroborated in the "objective" formulations of theoretical physics. When he looks through the eye of the scientist, he sees the evolutionary history of the universe as coherent in terms of scientific categories. When the same man looks through the eye of faith, he perceives the creative activity of God in both the order and the novelty of the whole dynamic web of interconnected events. The synthesis is seamless, not as a metaphysical system but as a personal faith, grounded in the purposeful creativeness of God. Drew summed it up:

> I think it comes down to a question of self-esteem. It's hard for people to feel—they feel unworthy to live in a universe where their life has purpose. It's a whole different way of looking at life, thinking that your life has purpose versus here you are, what do you do with the present situation? It's easier, you know, [to say] here I am, I'm too small to be noticed by God. It affects all your values.

That was the last sentence of our recorded conversations. In it, Drew identified the transformative belief, the one that "affects all your values." He believes that in a wondrously nonlinear way, God knows him and invests his life with purpose. This purpose implies no conventional, linear teleology—perhaps it is no teleology at all—but a trusting willingness to *go with the flow*, as the saying has it, even the turbulent flow of a chaotic system. The universe is hospitable not because there is a predetermined goal or future toward which it moves, according to plan, but because God's loving creativity can be discerned in the realization of the present.

That faith attitude is transformative across all his practices. Several of Drew's sentences from an earlier part of the conversations bring the attitude of his science-saturated faith into definitive focus:

> But chaos theory tells you that there's an expectation a lot of people will die in car accidents in 1995, but there's nobody walking around today who's "destined" to die in a car accident, because those decisions leading up to that car accident haven't been made yet. [It is] truly obvious that you can't decide today what you're going to believe tomorrow, or do. Which is why I believe Christianity is not a leap of faith; *it's a leaping of faith.* You can't decide today what you're going to believe tomorrow!

Conclusions

The conversations with Drew did not end with a solution to the problem of evil but with the doxology of a faithful man, amazed all the more by the majesty and mystery of the Creator because of his practice of science. The feature that distinguishes a pastoral or other clinical situation from a philosophical argument is that we are dealing with embodied persons, not disembodied ideas. What form does truth take when it is mediated by a life, or by a practice? Persons embody patterns of experience and interpret them into narratives that give them a point of view from which to see and act in the world. Drew, grounded in his particularity, unschooled in theology or philosophy but educated in science and business, experiences a "leaping of faith" that probes, synthesizes, and persistently embraces life as it comes to him with wonder, love, and praise. The narrative we created together is a testimony to that faith attitude—Drew's truth.

Yet, it is an attitude informed by reason. Meanings are communicated by these conversations. It would not stretch Drew's truth to observe that God functions as Cocreator of present and future reality, with Drew and the rest of humankind being the other actors in the process of creation. God, *Creator Spiritus* in the conversations, is not best understood as an omnipotent agent who decides and controls either natural or historical events. We know God in the awareness of a "seamless" presence who is with us through all happenings, even injustice. We withdraw from defining *how* God is present in the world. Because we are only now emerging from the Newtonian box of linear rationality, none of us knows our way around a perceived world of multifactorial, nonlinear processes well enough to find exact metaphors for divine action. Yet Drew, as an informed scientist and reflective Christian, has articulated some cosmological assumptions in this conversation that indicate promising pathways for explor-

ing the theological question more fully. I have suggested that Drew's illuminating phrase, *leaping of faith*—which, with the rest of his conversation, is consistent with a process theism that understands the human as cocreator with God
of an undetermined future—is such a pathway.

The role of chaos theory in opening this scientist's faith in God is another
pathway. Chaos theory is a relatively new paradigm in scientific thinking. Chaotic systems are composed of linear, cause-and-effect processes but generate unpredictable behavior because of the exponential amplification of uncertainties
in the initial conditions. The system as a whole, therefore, is nonlinear and indeterminate as to course, like weather systems or the marketing and service systems
Drew works with daily. Drew finds chaos theory pertinent for grasping and ar-
ticulating his convictions that the present and future are open, that God is actively with us in them, and that it is not God's will that "causes" events such as
the birth of a severely handicapped child. Other scientists and theologians have
explored how chaos theory may or may not be useful in asserting a
nondeterministic universe.[3] Drew shows how it translates into personal faith.

Simple cause-and-effect thinking—what most of us regard as common rationality—cannot explain God's connection with events we consider evil, any more
than such thinking is adequate to account for causality in any complex system.
Nancy's question, "Why did God let this happen to me?" was framed by her
assumptions of God as Monarch exercising mechanical causality and control in a
Newtonian universe. Could the chaplain help her not only to express her anger
and bewilderment, arguably the most immediate pastoral task, but also to reframe
her question in terms of a cosmology that has trust and creativity, rather than
causality and control, at its core? Could she be helped to ask, for example, in her
own way, the question formulated by James Gustafson,[4] "What is God calling
and enabling me to be and to do in this situation?" or that proposed by William
F. May,[5] "How shall I rise to the occasion?" Thus another conversation begins,
this time with Nancy, and more narrative data is generated that may help us tell
the truth about God and human suffering.

In addition to these theoretical pathways suggested by Drew's conversation, a
methodological conclusion is also pertinent to clinical practice. I have used a
simple method called biographical conversation and claimed that it leads to narrative truth. Conversation *per se* does not produce a narrative. The conversation
is interactive, intersubjective, and spontaneous, following the impulses of ideas,
memories, connections, and feelings. Conversations are as nonlinear and multifactorial as life. The narrative summary quoted in this paper represents a process
of "grasping together," in Paul Ricoeur's terminology,[6] the multiple elements of
the conversations into a coherent, sequential account—analogous to the interpretive process by which one makes meaning out of the flux of one's life. The role
that I as conversation-partner play in the process is to model interpretation by

doing it, offering the model back to the subject for criticism. Does the model "fit"? In other words, does my interpretation align with yours? Does it encourage you to be an active interpreter of your life and practices? Does it carry forward the conversation by evoking new perceptions or insights?

This evocative function of the method may be seen in the conversation with Drew. It was I, not he, who made explicit the connection between his affinity with chaos theory and the presence in his home of a severely handicapped son. I did so by suggestion in the initial conversations, then reiterated the connection in the narrative summary that I gave him to read. Drew and his wife were "somewhat rattled" by my references to their son. In a personal communication from Drew's wife, they carefully reemphasized how loving their son is and how much he appreciates life, continuing in this vein:

> [We] both thought that since you were interested in how our son is part of the family, you or your readers may be interested in our daughter, too, especially since she came to us also in an unusual way. Partly because I have to be home for [our son], but also because Drew and I both felt that we could provide a home for a child who really needs one, we got into foster care. . . . We got our daughter when she left the hospital at the age of 2.5 months. Due to her birth history she was at risk for problems and was on a monitor, but compared to [our son] she was in good shape. She has been with us ever since, and we adopted her when we were allowed to do so, just after she turned 4 years old. If you choose to [include] in your paper the reference to her advent into our home, we are hoping that the alert reader will realize that not only do we accept and appreciate our son, whom we never would have chosen to be so handicapped; we actively sought out another child with a difficult beginning and a very uncertain future, just because a baby needs and deserves a home and a life.

My original narrative summary contained no reference to their daughter. I rewrote it, as it appears now, to bring out the fuller dimension of their practice of parenthood and, in doing so, discovered through the tension itself an even deeper connection between Drew's relationship with his children and his appraisal of physical and spiritual reality. Perhaps we both became clearer about what it means to be a cocreator with God, and to move with trust, conviction, and action (such as the adoption of an at-risk child) into a future that is radically open. Thus, the conversation continues and the narrative evolves as meanings are shared, deepened, and incorporated. That, I believe, is the way truth takes form when mediated by a life.

5

Someone Is Always Playing Job

Margaret E. Mohrmann

Perhaps the best-known lines in Archibald MacLeish's play *J.B.* are these: "If God is God He is not good. If God is good He is not God. Take the even, take the odd."[1] The play is a twentieth-century version of the biblical story of Job, and these lines are chanted, like a child's rhyming game, by the character who represents Satan during an angry conversation with the character portraying God. The lines, like much of the rest of the play, can initiate a discussion of the formal question of traditional theodicy: Given the existence of evil in the world—or, in some formulations, given the excessive amount of evil—is it possible to believe that God is both entirely good and omnipotent (the attribute implied by the phrase "if God is *God*")?

This is the metaphysical issue raised by a superhuman character in the play, but the questions asked by the human J.B., like those asked by the original Job, sound more like this: "Given what I believe—even *know*—to be true about God's power and goodness, how can I possibly understand the evil, the dreadful suffering that has come upon me and those I love? How can I now understand myself and my world in relation to God if this can happen to me?" It is a thesis of this chapter, and, I submit, of the three "clinical" chapters preceding this one,[2] that the questions asked by sufferers in the midst of their pain are much more like those wrung from the stricken heart of Job/J.B. than they are like the logical puzzles analyzed by many philosophers and theologians.[3] As Albert Keller says in chapter 4, "It is not the intellectual history of the question that impinges, but its immediate power to shape the sufferer's experience of the divine in her life and to frame her capacity to meet the present crisis. That is the reason I approach theodicy as a faith question, not as a philosophical conundrum."

For most persons suffering medical ills, it would appear, the puzzle is not the ancient and enduring theological problem of theodicy, but a present religious or spiritual dilemma. Religion (and spirituality), most broadly, denotes the more or less systematic construction of meaning, which may or may not find expression in the liturgies and doctrines of one or another religious organization. Religion is how one puts it all together—birth, love, work, sex, family, suffering, joy, death—and discovers or creates, within these recurring and universal experiences, patterns and interconnections that suggest purpose and order. The power of suffering to break patterns, to confound carefully wrought and tenderly nurtured ideas of identity, relationship, and place in the cosmos can make it the occasion of spiritual crisis. But, even for the person whose spirituality is deeply theistic, the questions arising from this crisis are often not theological, but religious—questions not about how God may be defined, but about how previously understood patterns can be reconceived so that they may once again supply spiritual sustenance and hope.

This chapter, therefore, is about theodicy, but not theodicy as analyzed by the theologian seeking to justify God, or even to make God plausible, in the face of manifest evil. It is about theodicy heard in the queries and groans of sufferers and enacted in the ministrations of those who care for them, theodicy that, within certain understandings of God, seeks to comprehend the evil of the suffering that presents itself to medicine for relief, and to reweave meaning and order into the torn fabric.

The Nature of the Question

They were a young couple, confused and distraught. Their one-year-old son, Eric, was in the pediatric intensive care unit, on a ventilator, deathly ill with bacterial meningitis. I was the attending physician; I came by to have my usual twice-daily long talk with them about Eric's current status. After I had finished giving my report and answering their questions, we sat for a moment, silently mulling over the unknown future. Then Eric's mother said,

> I do have one other question. You've explained how the meningitis happened, but I still don't understand *why* he got it in the first place. Is it because there's something wrong with him? Or because I took him to the grocery store with me when he had a cold? *Why* did Eric get this terrible thing?

I thought then that she was asking unsophisticated questions about pathogenesis. I knew it was just chance whether a child picked up that particular bacterium, and another kind of chance whether it went on to cause meningitis. Immediately, there was on the tip of my tongue the sort of flip and savvy answer I had heard from my teachers and had myself quickly learned to foist on my students— "luck of the draw." But then I looked at her—I saw the entreaty in her eyes—and instead said, "I don't know. There's no reason to think there was anything unusual about Eric. We just don't know why some children get this and others don't." It was many years before I understood that she may have been asking, even without being fully aware herself of the scope of her question, about causality in a cosmic sense rather than in narrowly pathological terms.

David Morris, in *The Culture of Pain*, writes, "Humankind—across cultures and across time—has persistently understood pain as an event that demands interpretation. . . . It seems we cannot simply suffer pain but almost always are compelled to make sense of it."[4] Part of the process of making sense of pain and suffering, of the imposing presence of evil in our lives, is finding a way to seek that sense. What is the right question to ask, and to whom should it be directed? Is there some guide available for this task of interpretation? And what precisely is it that needs interpreting—the pain? that it exists at all? that it is afflicting me or this person I love (and, therefore, me also) specifically?

It is no wonder that the language adopted for the task of seeking understanding may not be explicitly the language of faith; the question may not mention God. My medical colleagues and I have to think long and hard to remember situations in which we were asked a question that sounded like a theodicy inquiry. Far more often the questions are narrowly practical, focused on the particular event, prefaced by the word "why." Like Eric's mother's queries, the question may sound "medical"—Why has this disease occurred in this person?—and susceptible to medical answers that use data about immunologic vulnerability or cumulative risk factors or hazardous lifestyle choices or, increasingly, genetic endowments.

Initial attempts to interpret suffering associated with afflictions identified as medical are often couched in a language appropriate for the specific disorder. And the resulting questions are asked of the person who seems most directly to have control over the disorder, the physician. It takes a sensitive, courageous ear to hear underlying concerns about God's power and goodness in relation to evil when the question being asked is, "Why did this disease happen to me?" Or, "I'm doing everything you recommended. Why don't I feel better?" Or, "Why haven't you doctors found a way to cure this yet?" Even if the clinician recognizes the spiritual "why?" that may lie behind the putatively medical "why?" how can she or he respond in a way that neither dismisses the literal question nor ignores the deeper anxiety?

I do not know if Eric's parents were consciously framing questions of cosmic significance, but I wonder if I could have helped them by going beyond my admission of ignorance to showing myself open to hearing what may have been their deep perplexity in the face of such a catastrophe. If the clinician receiving the question does not hear the cosmological undertones—whether because of inattention or inability or unwillingness—what then becomes of the patient's spiritual puzzle? Many physicians and, I suspect, many chaplains know that questions so difficult to formulate and so frightening to broach, similar to ones about the imminence of death, once deflected are in many cases never attempted again. Any implicit message, either about the impermissibility of such an inquiry or

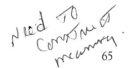

about the unavailability of the chosen interpretive guide, may be taken as a final
refusal of the possibility of finding or constructing meaning.

A friend told me a disturbing story about her father's dying. When it was made
clear to him that his death from cancer was imminent, he asked that his pastor
visit him, insisting that he had to talk with him as soon as possible. My friend was
there when the pastor came. Her father brushed aside the clergyman's greeting
and said urgently, "I must talk with you now." My friend began to leave, realizing
that her father might want privacy, but the pastor said heartily, "Oh, no, don't
go. Stay and we can have a nice visit." Her father frowned and said again, "No. I
need to talk with *you*, pastor!" The pastor's reply: "Now, now, nothing could be
that urgent. Everything will be fine. Let's just have a prayer, and I'll be on my
way. I don't want to tire you out." My friend took over from her weary and dis-
heartened father the task of importuning the pastor for the confessional ear she
thought her father wanted, but was no more successful than he. After the pastor
left, her father had little to say to anyone, refused to talk about his impending
death, and also refused any further visits from his pastor. Whatever the reasons
for the pastor's ignoring his parishioner's need, there was no one else to whom
the dying man chose to turn for the final peace he seemed to be seeking. This
story is about the failure of a clergyperson; it could as easily—perhaps more easily—be about a physician adamantly refusing a patient's desperate request to go
deeper into the great matters at hand, refusing the patient's need for a particular
companion for that perilous foray.

When we undertake that perilous work of making or finding sense in pain,
we begin with some conceptual framework for our thinking, a framework that
is usually so much a part of our cognitive apparatus as to seem unchosen and
often to go virtually unnoticed. For many physicians and for even more patients,
this interpreting matrix—the hermeneutical circle, if you will—includes some
idea of who God is and how God acts with us, and, therefore, of how the world
works. Our frameworks often contain deeply entrenched assumptions about God,
the kind that make it possible for MacLeish to say "if God is God" in the knowledge that his audience will recognize what is packed into that definition by identity.[5] It is in relation to our own cosmological framework that pain and suffering, of self or loved ones, has to make sense.

Listen to Julia Connelly's patient in chapter 3, asking, "Why me?" Her question is not "What's wrong with God that God would do (or allow) this?" She is
not calling God to account. She is placing herself in the dock—What's wrong
with *me*?—and searching for reasons within herself and her actions that can make
sense of such a fate in a world governed by the God she knows. Like Tolstoy's
Ivan Ilych,[6] she postulates a pathogenetic fall, but she goes further: "The devil
was there."[7] Obliquely she wonders if her smoking, even thirty years before, could

explain this affliction. Perhaps the illness was caused by the devil, or by her disobedient action, or by her occasional failures to care for her body. She does not ask if or why God may have inflicted this suffering; on the contrary, she finds a way to see it as, if not altogether just, at least a trivial injustice when compared to similar disease in a child. This nonanswer—which seems not to lead her to ask why the child is stricken—allows her to rest once again in her previous understanding of God's world, and to die in peace. It is as though, like Job, she was faced down by a blunt reminder of God's power (How could I "have been so bold to question God?"), and then supplemented that tacit rebuke by remembering her own long life and the evidences within it of God's goodness.

The near-dualism of this woman's framework—manifested in the role attributed to the devil—exemplifies what may be a widespread assumption, based on interpreted life experience, of a "dark side" to God. In *Birdsong*, Sebastian Faulks's riveting novel about the First World War, the main character uses an eclectic ritual of divination to reassure a comrade (Weir) about his fate in the forthcoming battle. He explains the strange activity to a new roommate: "This is voodoo I invented to pass the long hours. Weir likes it. It makes him feel that somebody cares about him. It's better to have a malign providence than an indifferent one."[8] Whether the malignity is thought to reside within God or within an equally, or almost equally, powerful devilish double, it seems that many people would rather assume that good *and* evil powers are somehow in control of the world, and that the balance between them shifts periodically, than believe that there is one all-powerful god who is "good" but nevertheless willing to allow creatures to suffer for no apparent reason. Dualism and belief in a cosmic struggle between the forces of light and darkness may be working theodicies that some find preferable to facing an abyss of apparent randomness and meaninglessness in which one's fundamental assumptions about God are untenable.[9]

Sometimes the search for meaning requires reconceiving God. The question then is still not the formal question of classical theodicy: In the face of this evil, how can one believe God to be the all-powerful, loving, utterly good deity proclaimed by countless generations of theologians and preachers? It is more a query about how a God so described could *also* be involved in evil. Listen in chapter 2 to the mother and aunt of Deborah Healey's imperfectly formed, and possibly molested, patient: "How can God do this to a child?" Included in that question is a prior assumption about who God is and how God acts, about all the attributes implied by the name "God." The task now is to make sense of this new information within that assumption.[10] We do not know how or if the family members resolved their question. But we do hear the physician's response: reception of and care for the spiritual distress, and guidance forward. The doctor claims no answer to the question about a possible causative role for God in the child's affliction, but does offer a response that, in practice, shows that God can be involved with them in their suffering.

Albert Keller's conversation partner Drew makes a statement that could have been given in reply to the questions asked by the persons presented by Connelly and Healey, as well as in reply to the reality of his own child's handicaps. Speaking of the nexus of indeterminacy and responsibility, Drew says, "It changes the way you look at life, and God's purpose, and where you think the interface is between God's will and your freedom of choice." This pinpoints the focus of the query as being not so much the nature of God as how God's nature—accepted, "known," often unquestioned—touches upon a particular instance of suffering. How can the God we experience in certain ways at times of joy and trust and clarity be involved, responsive, and responsible also at times of pain and struggle and confusion?

Construing the Issue

The title of this chapter echoes a line in MacLeish's play: "There is always someone playing Job."[11] It signifies that, in contemporary life, some person—probably many persons, of course—is always playing Job's role: the committed believer, stricken by physical, emotional, and/or social misfortune, who struggles to understand a conceptual world turned upside down. The challenge for the clinician—physician, nurse, chaplain, therapist—is to recognize this agonizingly puzzled figure in the person of the patient, to hear the cries of spiritual distress—the laments, protests, self-examinations—within the pressing attempts to grasp the nature and source of the disease and to control its course.

Stories and Tragedy

Clinicians hear the difficult, multilevel questions—about the way one understands life, about God's designs, about the interplay of divine and human roles in situations of suffering—always in the context of the patient's specific history and course of woe, relief, or relapse. Each of the three practitioners who contributed chapters for this book, having been asked to address the issue of theodicy as it arises within their professional experience, chose to rely on narrative. Dr. Healey tells a string of stories, each illustrating some way in which God is brought into the clinical encounter by and for her and her patients. Dr. Connelly emphasizes the importance of stories and scatters illustrative tales throughout her chapter. Reverend Keller constructs his conversational study on the thesis that relevant truth is mediated by a particular life, the recounting of which gives rise to insights unavailable except through narrative.[12] Focusing on the rubric of stories—and, even more specifically, on tragedy—seems a useful and truthful way to accomplish the work of recognition and reception that questions of God and suffering require.

Richard Selzer, surgeon and poetic observer of patients and doctors, has written that "to *perceive* tragedy is to wring from it beauty and truth," and thereby to approach the possibility of caring for one another.[13] Connelly's discussion of tragedy in relation to her patients, drawing on Larry Bouchard's writings on the subject[14] and corresponding to his chapter in this book, underscores the accuracy of Selzer's observation. As Bouchard and Connelly explain, tragedy involves not only suffering, but also critical choices—those that seem to have led to the disaster, those that may be scarcely remembered, those that must now be made, those that are now foreclosed—and the vertiginous experience of having crossed the limits of our ability to understand what is happening and why.

In the context of a practical, medical theodicy, the issue of choice can be heard in the sufferer's self-examination and self-blame. Questions of desert seem inescapable, in Connelly's chapter, for the mother who allowed her daughter to go out and must now deal with her death in an automobile accident, and for the woman with lung cancer who searches for culpability in her long-ago smoking and her more recent climb. Healey's patient Ann must grapple in the aftermath of rape with the decisions that led up to her presence in that motel room.

Choices, constrained by the tragic circumstances themselves, also become routes of survival and growth. Ann saves her own life by choosing not to abandon her mother, and perhaps salvages some of her conceptual world and some sense of worth by attributing that choice (and not the choices that preceded the assault, apparently) to God's attentive guidance. The decision, discussed in chapter 4, by Drew and his wife to adopt a potentially disabled child appears to have arisen from a sort of self-study occasioned by their son's affliction. Connelly's patient chooses, along with radiotherapy, an acceptance that seems to grant her a peace that no longer requires answers, a way of dying not fraught with her earlier anxiety and self-recrimination.

Of more immediate concern to the questions of theodicy than the issue of choice, however, is the matter of exceeding the boundaries of understanding. It is this, and not choice—the fact of choice, indeed, may at times be tried as an answer—that compels the question "why?" from the heart of one whose conceptual, spiritual cosmos no longer displays order or seems subject to benign governance. Because the experience of coming up against the limits of understanding is itself painful, it may be that the anxious spiritual questioning that can accompany suffering also increases the pain. If this is true and if relief of suffering is a primary goal of medical and pastoral intervention for the ill and injured, then attention to the patient's bewilderment may be as important as proper doses of analgesics or antidepressants are for subduing pain.

After detailing the evidence of medicine's general inattention to "the problem of suffering," David Morris turns to tragedy as a category that can refocus physicians' attention: "The question that tragedy poses to medicine is what to make of suffering. This is an inquiry that invites meditation and discussion rather than brisk true/false answers."[15] Tragedy seems to be understood rather widely, by lay people and health professionals, as a category with enough intrinsic meaning to be useful for making sense of a chaotic and painful situation; witness the effects of Connelly's use of the term on herself, her patients, and her coworkers.

To call a situation a tragedy seems to endow the events with a transcendent seriousness, while at the same time allowing, even requiring, them to exceed the limits of comprehensibility. Acknowledging that a patient's injury or loss or uncertain future or impending death is a matter of high dramatic significance grants permission for the patient's intense preoccupation with what is happening to him or her, and relative withdrawal from other matters that now seem shadowy and peripheral. Such recognition elevates the task of seeking understanding from the level of mere "fretting"—a label too often assigned to patient "complaints" by physicians, family, and, eventually, the patient—to that of solemn and respectable examination, contemplation, discernment, and decision.

Bouchard has said, "Awareness of tragedy probably 'solves' no formal moral question; rather, it encourages us to view the irresolvable character of some moral problems truthfully."[16] Facing the truth that some problems—medical as well as moral—cannot be resolved is the first step that both health care professionals and chaplains must take as they seek to bring relief to those who suffer. To claim or imply that medicine can solve (even someday) every physical source of pain and distress or that theology can answer (even mystically) every anxious query about God in relation to personally experienced evil is to turn away from the reality of suffering's too-often "irresolvable character." Patients whose physicians or chaplains give false, facile answers, which contradict the patients' lived experience and make their continued physical or spiritual distress merely a matter of their obstinate refusal to be comforted, cannot help but feel betrayed by the very persons who are supposed to be supporters and relievers, or, worse, betrayed by themselves in their inability to be quieted.

Wendy Farley, paraphrasing ideas expressed in the book she is reviewing, writes of the usefulness of the category of tragedy for theology; she could as well be speaking of its utility for medical practice:

> Tragedy, for Sands [the author reviewed], is a way of maintaining the openness of theology, disciplining it for a capacity to listen to the non-sense, the outside-of-sense of suffering. The rush for meaning that can amputate experiences irreducible to explanations is challenged.[17]

The "capacity to listen to the non-sense . . . of suffering" is a hard-won skill. For physicians, particularly, professional education is partly a process of weeding out "nonsense," of learning to give up for oneself, and to set aside when heard from one's patients, seemingly magical lay notions of disease etiology (Can one really catch cold from sitting in a draft?), natural history, and effective treatment (Do raw beef poultices really get rid of warts? Or copper bracelets draw out the pain of arthritis?) in favor of validated scientific explanations. Even simple pragmatism in the face of benign nonscience (If your arthritis hurts less when you wear copper bracelets, by all means wear them) may be rejected, although sometimes at the cost of credibility.

But the intensity of suffering is often directly related to its degree of senselessness.[18] The clinician who fails to attend to the non-sense aspect of suffering may miss precisely the critical spiritual issues at stake. To deflect the deepest "why?" questions, as though they were equivalent to inquiries about phlogiston or indictments of miasma, with the self-protective glibness of "Why not?" or, in my more usual idiom, "Luck of the draw," is to run from nonsense straight into meaninglessness—not a journey of growth, to say the least.

These last two answers, even when expressed with compassion and softened by euphemism, represent two effective and common methods of "amputation" of the experience of suffering and the search for meaning. The first—"Why not?"—while perhaps bearing its own provocative truth, serves only to thrust the question back at the sufferer, at the same time admonishing him or her for inappropriate temerity or insufficient humility. The equation of the sufferer with every other potential victim of such pain gives substance to the specter of randomness, and denies the uniqueness of both sufferer and suffering. Although it may squelch the questioning, and perhaps allow the clinician to feel some satisfaction with his or her own forthrightness, "Why not?" may only intensify suffering by heightening its meaninglessness. A reminder of cosmic unfairness does little to comfort an agonizing physical or emotional experience of that unfairness. And it would take a patient with more strength and courage than many have left in the midst of their pain to give the appropriate retort to "Why not?": "That's precisely my point, doctor: Why not you or someone you love or any other person you can name? 'Why not?' only restates my question; it doesn't answer it."

The second dismissive answer, "Luck of the draw," even more explicitly assumes randomness. With no reference to even the possibility of fairness, the phrase suggests a metaphorical metaphysical game of cards, without so much as a dealer, in which one is as likely to draw the ace of spades as the king of hearts. The physician may have already come to terms with the notion of cosmic gaming for herself or himself (although, for many, the remark may be more like whistling in the dark), but imposing an authoritative pronouncement of universal indifference in response to a patient's "Why?" may be a manifest violation of the ancient injunction to "do no harm."

The conscious invocation of the rubric of tragedy can serve to remind us, clinicians and patients alike, not only of the painful role that choice plays in the development and maintenance of suffering, but also of the crucial fact that, by definition, suffering reaches beyond the ability of sufferers (and onlookers and helpers) to understand. The clinician's embrace of suffering's characteristic non-sense may help avert a destructive truncation of the sufferer's search for meaning and order.

Everyday Tragedies

One important caveat about use of the category of tragedy, however, is that an emphasis on the generally salutary "elevation" of the patient's experience to the level of high drama by endowing it with the trappings of the tragic may, on the other hand, mean that we shall recognize tragedies only when they are played out in the arenas we associate with dramatic and complex medical crises—intensive care units, oncology wards, emergency departments, rehabilitation facilities. It is important that we hear, in the three preceding clinical chapters, the pervasive theme of "everydayness." There is always someone playing Job; the drama is acted out on all sorts of stages, everywhere, every day.

Connelly speaks not only of the woman facing cancer or the mother whose daughter was dead on arrival at the emergency room, but also of the "everyday ethical issues and everyday tragedies . . . embedded in the everyday life of the community." She wonders whether this very quality has diminished her recognition of various incidents as "tragedies" and, therefore, has kept her both from perceiving the depth of her patients' consternation and from offering the understanding and help she believes the category affords. Keller refers to Drew's, and his wife's, "everyday life" and "everyday faith" specifically in relation to their welcoming a second, possibly handicapped child into their family. But throughout Keller's conversations with Drew one can note that the profound questions that arise for many people only at a time of crisis are often uppermost in Drew's mind. One emphasized aspect of Drew's depiction of the cosmos is the subtle but critical importance of precisely the "everyday," the minute, unnoticed, perhaps unconscious acts and responses that are part of the nonlinear determination of our indeterminate futures. He, I suspect, would accept Connelly's patient's association of both her previous smoking and her more recent fall with her current affliction, not in the "scientific" sense (in the language of medical science's linear notions of cause and effect, that is) but in the sense that multiple, nonlinear connections among events affect and shape what might otherwise appear utterly random and disordered.

In Healey's chapter the quotidian nature of the stories she reports confronts us both with the dreadful prevalence of intense suffering and with the implied consequences of failure to recognize the tragic nature of the everyday lives of many people. It is too clear that she encounters these stories of abuse, despair, shredded hopes, and stunted lives almost daily in her practice—a practice that takes place in a primary care clinic, not an intensive care unit. It is also clear that intensive care is what she is called on to provide. Like recent novels describing the combined desperation and resilience that characterize life for many,[19] Healey's briefly told tragedies highlight all the ways in which ordinary people hurt each other and themselves every day. The pervasiveness of evil in her tales is almost overwhelming in its blunt reality, but we are enlightened—and reminded of the revelatory and cathartic values of tragedy—by her refusal to "explain" the evil, her choice to juxtapose the stories instead with experiences that reveal to her the equally compelling presence of good, her willingness to hold these fragments together (in the eloquent language of Bouchard's chapter in this book) in order to frame her healing responses.

Responding and Responsibility

Perhaps the first thing to say about the clinician's response to questions that seem to be about theodicy is that the response cannot be an answer in the usual sense of the word. Although the particular physician or nurse or chaplain may have a more or less satisfactory—or, at least, quieting—answer to the problem worked out for himself or herself, there is no reason to think that the solution will be compatible with the question as the sufferer understands it. As Douglas John Hall reminds us, there is a problem with answers being given by persons who, unlike the sufferers, "have not lived long enough with the questions."[20] Moreover, there is too great a risk that providing a ready-made solution will cut off the sufferer's necessary, and potentially healing, attempts to find meaning and resolution for her or his own uniquely existential experience. More honest and more helpful in the situation may be either the reply, "I don't know," or the spontaneous response so characteristic of the human reaction to that which is beyond our understanding: the slow shake of the head, back and forth, accompanied by three humming syllables, mmm-mmm-mmm, that somehow effectively express both bafflement and lament.

What is most painfully not known within the puzzle of the presence of suffering in our lives, the puzzle of theodicy, is what we can expect of God's sense of morality. On the one hand, there are scriptural reminders that God's idea of justice and goodness may not be quite the same as ours. In the fearful Psalm 50, the psalmist, after detailing human acts of iniquity, has God say, "These things you have done and I have been silent; you thought I was one just like yourself" (Psalms 50:21). God's ethical otherness is also stressed in this passage from Isaiah: "For my thoughts are not your thoughts, nor are your ways my ways, says the

Lord. For as the heavens are higher than the earth, so are my ways higher than your ways and my thoughts than your thoughts" (Isaiah 55:8–9).

On the other hand, there is a deep human need to understand our creation in the image of God as telling us something about the nature of God as well as about our own nature, a need to believe that there can be no great discordance between our most cherished and consistent notions of the good and what God holds to be good. That is, we expect God to be at least as moral as we are and God's moral difference from us to be in degree—God is morally *better*—but not in kind. George Macdonald, the nineteenth-century Scots preacher and popular novelist, summarized this human expectation in a confidently insistent epitaph for one of his characters: "Here lie I, Martin Elginbrod: Have mercy on my soul, Lord God; as I would do, were I Lord God, and you were Martin Elginbrod."[21]

We stumble and guess at the relation between our moral premises and God's. Nevertheless, many believers hold that somehow, despite the gulf of otherness, God will be with us when the time of trial comes.[22] One who believes that may then be shaken to the core when plunged into an abyss of suffering in which no trace of God's sustaining presence is detectable. To be able to respond to a patient's suffering—that is, to be *responsible to* the patient—can be to overcome, to transcend the experience of loss and isolation by making God present through our own ministering attendance. The remainder of this chapter is about enacting this kind of responsibility.

Receiving the Story

> The sternest wisdom of Greek tragedy may be that suffering cannot be shared: only witnessed. . . .
>
> Perhaps what medicine can profitably relearn from tragedy is a sense of awe, even reverence, at the extraordinary struggles it is sometimes called upon to attend. Pain on occasion becomes the site of encounters we can do nothing except witness in respect.[23]

Listen to the voices of clinicians who "witness in respect." Dr. Healey: "I can provide no answer . . . But, I can receive from them their confusion, their fears for Crystal and her future, their sense of helplessness and lack of control, even their anger. . . . She had shared with me her pain and I could hold it with her."

Dr. Connelly, in response to the mother's asking "Why?" about her daughter's death, replies by naming the event a tragedy, allowing the respectful solemnity of that label to draw together the frantic, searching questions into a narrative structure that carries the hope of meaning. In response to the woman who asks, "Why me?" she recognizes the question's significance, reflects it back to her patient, and receives the convoluted reply with sufficient attention to be able not only to

reproduce it later from memory for her chapter but, more important, to recall it
for guidance in the care of her patient's dying. Reverend Keller, eager to engage
in dialogue with his conversation partner about the implications of Drew's thought
for Keller's own work, recognizes that the story must go where Drew is taking it:
"It was not the time for narrowing down, however. He was thinking theologically." Keller's silent and respectful reception allows Drew to give his clearest
statements of how chaos theory informs his understanding of God in relation to
human responsibility and suffering. At the conclusion of the interviews, Keller
confirms Drew's ownership of his story by asking him to review the transcripts to
be sure the retelling has been faithful. Reception, reflection, review—all components of the respectful witnessing that is our obligation to suffering patients.

Keller suggests that a chaplain may be able to lead a sufferer who raises theodicy
questions to ask instead the questions that structure the thinking of James M.
Gustafson and William F. May: What is God calling and enabling me to be and
to do? How shall I rise to the occasion? The clinician, too, could consider these
queries, but perhaps a more patient-centered question to guide reception of and
response to the sufferer's story is, "What is going on?"[24] Keeping this inquiry in
mind as we hear stories of pain and anxiety may help us lead the patient, and
ourselves, to deeper levels of understanding. It may also help us expand our understanding of patients' sense of desert from narrow notions of self-blame to a
fuller idea of responsibility.

Accepting the Patient's Responsibility

It is important for the clinician to think in terms of his or her responsibility
(ability to respond) *to* the patient. It is also important for the chaplain or nurse or
physician to accept the patient's sense of responsibility (to self or God or the
cosmos) *for* the disease as a step out of passivity that may be a prerequisite for
being able to respond *to* one's own suffering. When a patient muses that smoking
thirty years ago may have resulted in lung cancer, or a parent wonders whether
taking a toddler with a cold to the grocery store may have induced meningitis, it
may not be the clinician's place to pronounce an easy absolution by denying the
connection outright. Such a denial is likely to miss the deeper point and could
well be met with the rejoinder, "No, doctor, you don't understand. I'm telling
you that I am taking responsibility for this illness." J.B.'s angry reply to the "com-
forter" who attempts to eliminate the possibility of guilt by claiming a universal
innocence based on ignorance makes the point clear:

> I'd rather suffer every unspeakable suffering God sends, knowing it was I that suf-
> fered, I that earned the need to suffer, I that acted, I that chose, than wash my
> hands with yours in that defiling innocence. Can we be men and make an irrespon-
> sible ignorance responsible for everything? I will not listen to you![25]

Taking responsibility is not always synonymous with taking the blame. It may be an acknowledgment that one can connect events in a loosely causal manner without assuming that "because I did A, now B has happened to me." It may be a declaration of integrity that accepts the interconnections of all the parts of one's life, actively overseen by oneself. Drew's description, in Keller's chapter, of the nonlinear, nonrandom indeterminacy of human life captures this idea well. If there is some definite, even if not clearly definable, way in which a "sneeze today . . . averts a tornado six months from now," we cannot truthfully say that an outing with a child has *nothing* to do with the child's eventual illness. Instead of quickly relieving the overtones of blame, we need to hear deeper undertones of responsibility, the voice of complex human tragedy sounding in the apparently uncomplicated question of causation.

A respectful witness honors the deep and prevalent human certainty that the afflictions that befall us and those we love do not come upon us passively, randomly, meaninglessly. It is not only that we *need* to see pattern and sense in their coming; it is that our undeniable feelings of responsibility for what happens to us reflect something true about the world and our relations to God within this world. As Drew says, "It changes the way you look at life, and God's purpose, and where you think the interface is between God's will and your freedom of choice." To receive the story of suffering as it is, rather than as we wish it were to ease our own anxiety, is to embrace the truth of human responsibility, to endow it with the respectful seriousness of tragedy, and to avoid foreclosing it from the possibility of meaning and hope.

Discovering/Creating Beauty

When the "art" of medicine is discussed, almost invariably the focus is on such matters as bedside manner, the skills of instilling hope and inspiring trust, of treating patients as whole persons. Important as these skills are, to confine the concept of art to them is to limit art's definition to craft or technique: artisanship. But art is also defined as the making or doing of things that have form and beauty. Especially in dealing with the thorny questions that surround the relation of God to instances of human suffering, this aspect of medicine's—and ministry's—art is good to remember.

The pain of apparently random affliction, of seemingly meaningless pain, lies, as we have noted, at least in part in its disorderliness. The world is turned upside down; all prior understandings of connection, causation, structure, security totter and fall. Relief of this kind of suffering requires a creative act of reconstruction, reordering the pieces—perhaps with some old ones left out, new ones added—to remake the unmade world, in Elaine Scarry's evocative and enduring language.[26] Restoration of shape and order, however now revised, to one's world seems to be the sine qua non of spiritual healing, and perhaps, therefore, of complete physical healing as well. Healing requires, in some fashion, the creation or discovery of form and beauty.

As we read in the three clinical chapters in this book, the beauty created or envisaged may take any of a number of forms. The physicist Drew's theodicy is "similar in at least one aspect to the biblical book of Job: Each ends not in a rational solution to the problem . . . but in an affirmation of beauty." The beauty, for Drew, is in the recognition that, despite the difficult interplay of elusive indeterminacy and inescapable responsibility, God's goodness and love are evidently at work:

> On top of all the unfairness in life, we're learning how to be compassionate. On top of all our limitations, we're learning how to be cared for. On top of all the uncertainty in life, we're learning how to trust, and we're learning responsibility and commitment when other people put their trust in us. We're learning how to forgive.

These are not the blind platitudes of a naive man. They are a hymn to the wise and fecund beauty of a divine order that can use apparent chaos as an ordering principle, sung by a person who grapples with the reality of order-in-chaos daily in his work and at home. "It's one of the true mysteries of life how something that is so unjust and so unfair can be so beautiful!" Drew holds the contradictory fragments of a fully embraced life together and pronounces the whole "beautiful." Far from hiding behind the category of "mystery" as a way to avoid considering the oxymorons of life, he resolves the enigma by incorporating it, keeping the paradoxes intact and lovely in their richness.

Much as Drew moves seamlessly from indeterminacy and chaos to paradoxical order and beauty, Julia Connelly begins with the sense-making beauty of tragedy and ends with the order-creating art of poetry. For Drew, the beauty seems discoverable by the mind prepared to enjoy the contrapuntal response of compassion to injustice, of commitment to limitation. For Connelly, in contrast, beauty is created by the mind seeking order, a process that may be heralded by questions like "Why me?" Although tragic events are tragic in part because they are experienced as random and past understanding, the category of "tragedy" can gather them into an art form that possesses its own classical sense of the cosmic and personal significance of human acts and their consequences. Tragedy holds the incommensurable fragments of choice, pain, responsibility, and helplessness in an embrace that imparts to them, taken together, meaning and a searing kind of beauty.

Poetry, on the other hand, seems, in Connelly's formulation, to be a different kind of art- and meaning-making. In the creation of poetry, the disorder is first allowed to fall apart again, out of tragedy's compass, into unrelated pieces that defy sense, so that the poet may "allow the disorder in." From experiencing the disorder as such, the poet may then begin translating it into language, whose particular forms and restraints impose a new order on the events.[27] Unlike tragedy, which displays the still-disordered events upon its formal backdrop, poetry transforms the painful chaos into the ordered limits of word and meter, sound and sense. Perhaps poetic transmutation of disorder can be seen as a "next step" in transcending serious suffering. That is, after the rubric of tragedy has served its purpose by keeping the events real and alive, providing a way to hold them together and present in tolerable perspective, then the act of making poetry of them produces the enduring beauty, the truly remade world.

Deborah Healey's evocation of art is somewhat different from Drew's and Connelly's. Like Drew, she includes a paean to the loveliness of God's love, the world, and human relationships; like Connelly, she wrestles explicitly with the physician's need to create form and beauty from the shattering stories with which she is faced. However, her "art" is woven throughout the tragic tales she tells, offering an immediate counterpoint of manifest goodness to the recurring ugliness of evil. This interplay, in contrast to summing or organizing themes, may be directly related to the nature of her medical work.

Healey's medical practice as both adolescent specialist and expert in child sexual abuse entails that she is confronted daily, even several times daily, by patients and families whose suffering is acute, severe, likely to be long-lasting and consequential, and not susceptible to usual—or even extraordinary—modes of medical treatment. Both for the healing of her patients and for her own survival as a sensitive, caring physician who is responsible to her patients, she must have immediate resources to counteract repeated and brutal manifestations of evil inflicted upon the relatively innocent for no apparent reason—the very stuff of theodicy's irresolvable dilemmas. Thus, as she recounts for us these dreadful tales, she constantly reminds herself and us of the other evidence available that God is indeed good, loving, and present. She begins with stories of patients for whom God is a partner in healing, a protector and haven in the midst of confusion and loss. Then she introduces patients or family members who ask "Why?" or who reforge with difficulty connections to a God who now represents their sole lifeline.

Only then, buried in the middle of the chapter, can she insert two horrific tales of evil perpetrated on children by the persons most responsible for them. In the context of these two stories, she must deal with her own issues of theodicy. Besides being present for the stricken patients and families, she must take care of herself and her students as they confront the enormity of humanly perpetrated evil written on the bodies and in the eyes of the children they are examining. The doctors must, after all, not only care for these patients, but also come back the next day to do it again for other patients who need their expertise and empathy. Healey explains, in introducing these stories, the importance of staying open to the horrors:

> After ten years of doing this work, I am in no way used to hearing the stories, and I have not become numb to my patients' pain. It is quite the contrary. I feel very directly for them and believe that, in order to provide compassionate care, I must be open to hearing just how bad things have been. Becoming numb might protect me in the short term, but it would also prevent me from forming any intimate connection with the family. I must be touched by the stories if I am to be an effective physician.

To be touched but not destroyed by the stories requires significant inner resources. For Healey, these resources are encapsulated as her faith, and this acknowledgment leads her on—and out of the dreadful stories—to evidences of God's love and goodness in her life *and* in her work.

It is the times of "connection," the "moments of grace" in Healey's practice that are an important sign to her of God's presence and love. Although she seems to accept an Augustinian definition of evil as the privation of good—"the complete absence of God and God's goodness"—she nevertheless has a strong sense of God's *presence* with her in situations where the consequences of evil are manifest. It is but a small step further to say that, by her constant awareness of God's presence—or, at times, her conscious efforts to invoke or regain that presence—and by her readiness to connect with her patients and families, Healey enables God's presence in these situations of dire suffering. Her practice, offered in *response* to the question "why?" (whether posed by the patient or by Healey herself) is also an *answer* to the question "Where is God in all this pain?": God is here with me; I am here with you; so God is here where the pain is.

Doing Theodicy

The "moments of grace" that Healey describes—like Connelly's specific invocations of tragedy and the creation of poetic order, and like Drew's astonished pleasure at cosmic beauty outshining injustice—are, as Bouchard says in his chapter, "also moments when theodicy occurs." Theodicy, in these chapters and in the practicing lives of health care professionals and pastors who minister to the ill, is practical, experiential, and paradoxical. It is less the abstract reconciliation of propositions about God, more the work of making things of form and beauty out of lived anxiety and pain. Elsewhere in this book, Nelson suggests that the vocation of medicine is an effective and revealing reply to the secular problem of evil because it allows its practitioners to work against evil in significant ways, while still preserving themselves and their individual modes of life. Similarly, the vocation of caring for the sick and injured responds to the theological problem of evil, the conundrum known as "theodicy," by allowing its practitioners to _be_ a way in which God's goodness and God's power to comfort and transform can be manifestly present despite the suffering.

Bouchard's idiom of "holding fragments" seems especially appropriate for the stories related in these chapters. The fragments cannot be knit together by reason to form, or reform, a meaningful whole. This fact is what makes the category of tragedy, which accepts the incomprehensibility of the "destructive _entanglements_ of innocent contingency and moral culpability," so useful and illuminating for retaining the disjointed pieces in their real, incommensurable, fragmentary form. But, as Bouchard insists:

> By "holding fragments," I do not mean being irrational, for to think with the fragments requires critical reasoning and assessment. . . . But I do mean to leave incomplete the bridges of thought between the stories, images, or actions we juxtapose. What now traverses the distance between the fragments may simply be the living, working, and abiding with others, even in the distances that separate us. What crosses between lamentation, solidarity, and protest may be attentive silence, or the recital of a psalm, or—as here—the stories of those who have also held fragments.

"Attentive silence," a moment of connection between physician and patient, a hymn to God's beauty _anyway_, wrestling the pain into poetry may all be modes of "doing" theodicy by and on behalf of those who suffer and those who care for them.

My patient Sarah, a nine-year-old girl with leukemia, was slowly dying in her isolation room in the intensive care unit. Her mother Joan sat silently with her all through each day as the child slept, or moaned, or roused to speak. For hours each day also, Agnes, the social worker who had known the family for several months, sat with them. With fond, puzzled amusement, Joan later told me—for years it was the only story she _could_ tell about those hopeless days—that Agnes was generally silent during her visits. But, every fifteen or twenty minutes or so, she would sigh, shake her head, and murmur, "I don't know." Nothing more. Joan smiled at this odd behavior, but it was clearly the only token from that terrible time she chose to hold on to; it meant something to her. I believe Agnes was "doing theodicy" with her honest lament, intoning the only phrase that, along with her caring, human presence, could hold together the fragments of Joan's and Sarah's lives—their hopeful past, their painful present, their unthinkable futures. Not understanding, but presence and truth, may help the unbearable somehow be borne.

Part 2

Theological Views

6

Finitude, Freedom, and Suffering

Daniel P. Sulmasy

Theodicy is an enormous, complex, and difficult enterprise. Even if the field of inquiry is limited to justifying or defending persistent belief in the loving good-ness and power of God in the face of *medical* suffering, the task is far greater than anyone can hope to accomplish in a brief chapter. Yet the task could not be more urgent. The questions of theodicy are not irrelevant at the bedside.[1] The con-temporary cry for legalized physician-assisted suicide and euthanasia might be considered a response, in part, to a lack of any credible medical theodicy; suicide may be the only reasonable alternative to medical theodicy.

I want to make clear that I am *not* treating theodicy as a synonym for natural theology, but as the justification or defense of belief in God despite the existence of evil in the world. Even more narrowly, I shall address *medical* theodicy, which I take to be the question of whether the following set of propositions can be asserted without contradiction:

1. God is all-powerful.
2. God is all-loving.
3. God is all-knowing.
4. God is the creator of all that is.
5. Human beings suffer through illness, injury, pain, and death.

Many have claimed that these propositions cannot be asserted as a unified set without self-contradiction. Persons have lost their faith in God in the face of their own illnesses or those of loved ones. Others have refused to believe in God because they cannot see how anyone could believe that God created human beings, loves us, and yet allows us to suffer the horrors of disease, injury, and death. At varying levels of sophistication, these issues face patients and clini-cians every day.

In this chapter, I hope to clear away some of the logical questions surrounding the problem of theodicy, questions that are appropriate to ask but are perhaps not too clearly answered. My goals are modest: I propose a *defense* of belief in the existence of God in the face of medical suffering. I do not propose a *justification*. That is, I simply argue that belief in God is compatible with acknowledgment of the reality of medical suffering, but I do not attempt to *justify* or *explain why* God should allow medical suffering. I want only to say that, in the end, the problem of medical theodicy is not a *logical* problem, and that I can support this conclusion by means of a logical argument. Patients raise the question, "How can God truly love me, truly be God, and allow me to suffer like this?" They suggest by this question that the above propositions are logically contradictory. If it can be shown that these propositions are not truly contradictory after all, it would be important for health care professionals and pastors to know this. Not only might they help patients avoid fruitless worry over the logical aspects of this question, but they might also be able to help patients focus on the important spiritual issues at stake.

The literature is filled with a variety of terms to classify various kinds of evil. It is therefore important that I be clear about how I define my terms. In this chapter, I use the term "material evil" to refer to all evils of the natural, physical sort, such as earthquakes, physical pain, and death. I use the term "moral evil" to refer to those actions or omissions that are deemed blameworthy failures of knowledge, will, affect, or love.[2] Some moral evils cause material evils (as when a mugger beats a victim), but there are many others that do not result in material evils (as when a family member refuses ever to communicate with another family member). Moral evil can cause physical evil because free human decisions affect the material world. However, if humans are truly free, the material world cannot directly control free human decisions. Therefore, material evils may tempt individuals to commit moral evils, but can never actually cause moral evils. Theodicy must account for both types of evil.

Is Theodicy Itself an Evil Enterprise?

Some persons argue today that attempting theodicy does more harm than good. Tilley, for example, claims that theodicy is a "discourse practice that ought to be abandoned," and that to engage in such a language game in the face of human suffering is both an insult to those who suffer and a distraction from attempts to relieve that suffering. Theodicy is an "opiate of the people" and an evil enterprise.[3]

But one must be clear about the aims and limits of theodicy. Theodicy makes no claim to be a bedside technique of *direct* assistance to the physician and the chaplain. It is as unfair to demand that theodicy do this as it is to demand that a scientist studying the kinetics of the reverse transcriptase enzyme of the human immunodeficiency virus (HIV) demonstrate the immediate clinical relevance of that work. The task of basic science research is understanding, not treatment.

The task of theodicy is understanding, not pastoral comfort. Those who engage in research, scientific or theological, may hope that better understanding of fundamental questions will eventually lead to better care, but the connection between research and care is neither immediate nor guaranteed. This does not mean that these enterprises are pointless.

On the other hand, no one should be deluded into thinking that fundamental questions are not relevant at the bedside. Each believing patient confronts the problem of evil in a unique fashion, plucked from the manifold ways in which illness, injury, and death can afflict the children of God. Each honest believing patient inevitably asks questions: Why has God allowed me to suffer from this disabling stroke? From the ravages of AIDS? From this debilitating rheumatoid arthritis? From this painful cancer? It is just as arrogant to suggest that they are asking the wrong question—and that theology must correct their primitive religious consciousness—as it is to respond with pious platitudes that fail to acknowledge the reality of their suffering.

Tilley suggests that theodicy is a misplaced enterprise because it is apologetic, directed toward nonbelievers, while the questions of theodicy are raised only by believers, who can be persuaded to "let go of" their questions by other means within a discourse community of faith. However, this presumes that the discourse communities of believers and nonbelievers are mutually exclusive and that questions of theodicy raised by believers have nothing in common with questions raised by nonbelievers. This seems quite odd. Whether asked in Latin or English, by believers or nonbelievers, the question seems to be whether or not there is a logical contradiction in a set of propositions. As long as there are persons who raise this question and find it a stumbling block to faith, theologians and philosophers of religion have an obligation to examine it. As Stanley Hauerwas observes, even if a patient raises the theodicy question in anger and in doubt, the asking is a very good thing.[4] It presumes a relationship with the God toward whom the anger and doubt are directed. A pastor might not read Hick, Swinburne, or Augustine to such a patient, but knowing what these theologians have said may help that pastor find something other than pious platitudes to offer. The questions of theodicy cannot be dismissed as irrelevant or misdirected from the perspective of suffering patients and their loved ones.

Being rational about suffering and faith is not evil, nor is making clear and logically precise arguments incompatible with being kind and compassionate. Kindness toward patients or other persons who ask questions about the world in a logical fashion and who want as much logical clarity as possible seems to require the use of logical analysis.

Theology cannot be antirational. Distrust of the sufficiency of reason to answer all theological questions does not imply that reasoning about God is inappropriate. For the believer, talk of God is not talk of nonsense. This is not to deny that there are aspects of God and of God's activity that surpass human understanding. But, whatever can be said of God ought to be compatible with what else is known about the world. If it is not, then what we think we know either about God or about the world must be re-thought. God's power and goodness and the existence of human suffering have to be shown not to be contradictory. If they are, then belief in one term or another must be mistaken.

Theology must be speculative. If theology is truly faith seeking understanding, then it must seek to understand. The pastoral implications of any theology need to be drawn out carefully, but the primary purpose of theology is understanding, not homiletics or pastoral counseling. Good homiletics and good pastoral care depend on a solid grasp of theology's understanding. Therefore, it seems critical for ministers, as well as for believing health care professionals, that speculative questions about the rationality of belief in God's loving goodness in the face of medical suffering be addressed.[5]

Theodicy is not evil. Ignoring the legitimate questions of theodicy may be.

The Classical Theodicies

Historically, there have been many attempts to answer the general question of how God could have all the attributes that believers have ascribed to God and yet allow so much evil in the world. Some answers are less satisfactory than others. I shall briefly describe and classify some of these arguments in order to situate my thinking in relation to prior work. I recognize, of course, that it takes more than a paragraph to do justice to any of these theories, but space does not permit detailed arguments.

Privation Theories

Privation theories are the classical theories regarding evil as articulated by Augustine,[6] Aquinas,[7] and Leibniz.[8] The basic thesis of the privation school of theodicy is a wonderful expression of Christian belief in the goodness of creation. Authors in this school assert confidently that God created a wholly good universe, but that there is a hierarchy in that universe. "Higher" beings have more good than "lesser" beings. Because of this, they conclude, evil is really an absence of goodness. In other words, evil has no positive existence; there is only a lack of good. While this view is interesting, many have found it less than satisfactory.[9]

Proving-Ground Theories

The approach of "proving-ground theories," attributed to Irenaeus[10] but fully developed only in the twentieth century,[11] offers an interesting alternative to

Augustinian theodicy. These theories do not deny that evil has real existence in the world, but hasten to add that it serves God's greater plans for humankind. God ordains that human beings should experience trials in this world as a way of helping us use our freedom to grow in wisdom, virtue, and grace. Quoting Keats, they urge that the world can be understood as a "vale of soul-making." The trials of the world are opportunities for learning charity, courage, and self-discipline.

While this theory has much to recommend it, many find it also inadequate. It is a rather anthropocentric view,[12] and it is at least problematic to suggest that the *purpose* of evil is human moral development.

Process Theology Approaches

Process theology has, to some extent, "solved" the problem of theodicy by denying the first proposition of the set, that God is all-powerful.[13] The God of process theology "persuades" the "actual entities," but exerts no true causation. Evil is contained within the panentheistic reality of God. This God enters into human history and can walk with human beings in their suffering. God can suffer with and for human beings and has done so historically through the life, ministry, passion, and death of Jesus Christ. But God does not cause evil and God does not remove evil. Evil is part of what is, part of what God, who fills the universe in all its parts, participates in by necessity.

This certainly solves the problem of evil. God is powerless to stop it, so there is no logical contradiction in God's "allowing" it. The problem, of course, is that many find it hard to imagine that this is the true God of Judaism and Christianity. It is sometimes suggested that the God of process theology may avoid the problem of evil but does not seem to be a god worthy of worship.

Existentialist Approaches

It has become fashionable, particularly given the inadequacies of other attempts at theodicy, to say that reverential silence before the mystery of human suffering is all that is possible.[14] Suffering cannot be explained. Those who ask for an explanation are themselves suffering from residual post-Enlightenment rationalism, asking questions that should not be asked, or from "poor theology" that forces them to conceive of these questions as consisting, at least in part, of important logical puzzles.

Those who hold this existentialist view argue that suffering is an unexplainable mystery that can only be pointed to by narrative and myth, forms of expression that do not arrogantly presuppose the possibility of rational explanation. The mystery of suffering is part of the mystery of God. The only "answer" one can give is found in an encounter with the mysterious loving presence that is always with us, even in our suffering. We need only place our trust and hope in this loving presence.

This approach has much to recommend it. It is often, I suspect, a very good pastoral approach. Saying the wrong thing about suffering at the bedside of a very sick patient can be very damaging; empathetic silence may be more effective. The approach has a truly "religious" (as opposed to "theological") character as well. It is more or less the answer God gave to Jesus in Gethsemane—mysterious, awesome silence.

Yet, as I stated above, the task of theodicy is not an immediately pastoral one. It is an enterprise in theology or in the philosophy of religion. It seeks an explanation, or at least a defense, of the compatibility of belief in God and the existence of evil. An appropriate answer might require mythic elements and take on an existentialist character, but more is required than the simple assertion that suffering is a mystery, no matter how good a story one tells about it.

In addressing the inexplicable, one must be careful to distinguish mystery from absurdity. Theodicy must at least explain why the existence of human suffering should not be an obstacle to faith. Camus, for instance, in his novel *The Plague*, tells a moving story of mythic proportions about human suffering.[15] But Camus takes suffering to be an absurdity, not a mystery, and counts the absurdity of suffering as a reason not to believe in God. Theodicy must give an answer to Camus, and to anyone else who thinks seriously and critically about God and illness. If belief in God in the face of human suffering is a contradiction, and suffering is real, then both suffering and theistic belief are absurd. But, if belief in God is defensible, even if not rationally explicable, in the face of human suffering, then it is possible to say that suffering is a mystery. To refuse to examine the logical aspects of the question is to abdicate an important mission for theology and the philosophy of religion.

Plantinga's Free-Will Defense

Alvin Plantinga has offered a clear, tightly argued defense of the compatibility of belief in God and the existence of evil.[16] Humbly, and in a manner that should assuage some of the complaints made against theodicy by the existentialist school, Plantinga does not offer an *explanation* of evil. He sets out to argue only that belief in a God who is the all-powerful, all-good, all-loving, and all-knowing creator of the universe is compatible with the existence of evil in the world. In brief, Plantinga's argument is that human beings with significant moral free will are better than human beings without such free will, and that it is at least possible that God could not have created a universe with genuine moral good (i.e., freely chosen good) that did not also contain moral evil.

Without going into the exacting detail with which Plantinga makes this argument, I shall simply say that I find it basically convincing as a defense of the compatibility of theism and *moral* evil. I have only two objections, the second more serious than the first. My first objection is that Plantinga argues that "transworld depravity" is essential to the nature of human beings, and that this is why natural necessity precludes the possibility of free will without evil choices. This premise plays an important role in his argument, and something like it is needed to make his argument work. My complaint, however, is that this premise is more acceptable to Calvinists than to Roman Catholics and, while I respect the Calvinist position, it is not my own.[17] Fortunately, because I find much value and insight in Plantinga's argument, I do not think the notion of "transworld depravity" is necessary for his argument to work as a defense of the compatibility of theism with moral evil. All that is necessary is to accept the premise that human beings are essentially morally fallible, a thesis closer to a Roman Catholic understanding of the human condition. Belief in total human depravity is not necessary, so a Roman Catholic can accept the premises of Plantinga's argument with only a minor adjustment.[18]

The second, more serious objection is that, while it seems that Plantinga's argument works for moral evil, it does not work well for material evil. In a chapter on medical theodicy, this could be a very serious deficiency. It would mean that belief in God is compatible with the horrors of moral evil committed by a Dr. Mengele, but that the theory does nothing to reconcile belief in God with the reality of suffering caused by malarial parasites, heart attacks, or broken hips.

Plantinga treats material evil only briefly, arguing that it is really a form of moral evil, ascribed to nonmoral persons (i.e., the fallen angels or devils). For Plantinga, malaria, angina, and crippling fractures are the consequences of Satan's abuse of Satan's own freedom. As a general rule, ad hoc additions to theories render those theories less probable, and should be avoided where possible. As Swinburne has pointed out, Plantinga's explanation seems quite ad hoc.[19]

Plantinga seems to suggest that the belief that material evil is caused by the fall of the devil is a fundamental tenet of Christian dogma. Nonbelievers, he suggests, might find it quaint, but believers ought readily to accept it. Certainly this story has been told throughout the centuries and might seem to be a deeply embedded, orthodox Christian teaching. But this is not the case. The theological justification for believing that Satan's sin is the cause of earthquakes and amyotrophic lateral sclerosis is really quite thin. Scriptural justification is largely apocryphal, with only two obliquely relevant references that attribute the existence of "death" to the devil (Wisdom 2:24, Hebrews 2:14). It is not at all clear whether these passages refer to moral or physical death. The Roman Catholic Catechism states only that the faithful believe that devils are angels who sinned; it attributes to the sin of these bad angels no material consequences for the physical universe.[20] Thus, the charge that an argument relying on such premises is ad hoc seems justified, because there is no strong dogmatic reason for such belief.

Such an assumption merely displaces the question onto Satan and does not advance the justification or defense of the compatibility of theism and material evil.

A Metaphysical Defense of Material Evil

One striking feature of all theodicies has been the tendency to recognize the meaningfulness of the distinction between material evil and moral evil and then to search for a single justification or defense that covers both. This strategy is pervasive, yet there is no logical reason or fundamental theological assumption that would require that there be one solution to cover both problems. Thus, the possibility remains open that a defense like Plantinga's may be adequate in the case of moral evil, but that some other sort of argument can be applied to material evil.

As stated above, the real problem in medical theodicy is material evil. Fortunately, the Dr. Mengeles among us have been few. Although greed, pride, sloth, and a host of other moral evils may plague the medical profession, and although the existence of such evils requires reconciliation with belief in a loving God, the fundamental problem for medical theodicy is not moral evil but material evil. I shall, therefore, spend the rest of this chapter presenting a preliminary sketch for a metaphysical defense of the problem of material evil as it is encountered in medicine. I see this approach as parallel to Plantinga's free-will defense of moral evil. Just as the good of free will is the capstone of Plantinga's defense of moral evil, so the good of creaturely existence is the capstone of my defense of the existence of material evil. The two may together constitute a defense of the compatibility of theism and the existence of all the evils encountered in the practice of medicine.

Being Human

Space does not permit a complete defense of an admittedly controversial basic point of view, but I shall at least identify my position regarding human beings as belonging generally to a school of thought that has been called "essentialist." I do not believe that any acceptable account of human suffering can be constructed without some notion of what human beings really *are*, without an account of human essence.[21] Nonetheless, the essential human characteristics I think are important in a discussion of human suffering are so basic that they are unlikely to be disputable, so those who are put off by essentialist views should press on. The set of species characteristics I list can be accepted as true of human beings even by those who would not agree that there is anything that could be called a human essence.

First, Judaism and Christianity hold that human beings are creatures. That is, we have been created by a God who is worthy of worship—all-powerful, all-knowing, and all-good. Human beings are made, not begotten, and are not one in being with God.

Second, it is clear that human beings are materially constituted. Human beings have human bodies; we are not created as disembodied spirits. Corporeality is an essential characteristic of human beings.

Third, it is characteristic of human beings that we have consciousness. I mean by this an awareness of self and environment that is more than mere biological arousal. This consciousness displays itself in a variety of ways—rational, emotional, imaginative, aesthetic, spiritual, and other modes. There may be individual members of the species who do not possess this characteristic, but it is nonetheless an attribute of the human. Severe diminutions in the level of consciousness or intellectual function of an individual member of the species *Homo sapiens* are not grounds for excluding that individual from the species. Those human beings who do not possess the species characteristic of consciousness are considered ill. To deny that permanently unconscious members of the species *Homo sapiens* are truly *human* begs the question of theodicy, because alterations in consciousness are counted among the physical occasions of human suffering that theodicy must explain or defend.

Fourth, it is characteristic of human beings that we are free. Catholic Christians believe that God has created human beings as essentially free in a significant way with respect to moral choices. This assumption of freedom is one that many people, not only theists, are willing to make. It cannot be fully defended in this space, but it is an important characteristic of human beings that, as Plantinga has pointed out, figures prominently in the justification of belief in God in a world characterized by evil. Things may go awry for some human beings with respect to their exercise of freedom, but those who never will possess freedom of choice or have at some point lost this freedom, through either human action or natural calamity, have suffered either moral or material evil. This freedom also cannot be denied in an argument about theodicy without begging the question, because being denied freedom is one of the ways in which human beings are said to suffer. The existence of a loving, all-powerful God and the existence of such suffering are two propositions that must be shown to be compatible if both are to be believed.

Fifth, it is characteristic of human beings that we have intrinsic dignity. This means that human beings have a meaning or value that is inalienable and depends only upon being human.[22] Christians believe this dignity comes from being created in the image and likeness of God.

Finally, it is characteristic of human beings that we are finite. Since there can be only one actual infinity (namely, God), human beings, as creations of the Infinite One, must be finite.[23] God can create only finite, fallible creatures.

Suffering and Being Human

The essential finitude of human beings expresses itself in at least two ways: morally and materially. As finite moral beings, human beings are essentially finite (fallible) in our moral choices. Only God is morally perfect. Human beings are also finite (fallible) in our reasoning abilities and nonmoral judgments. After all, "we're only human." The same is true of the physical nature of human beings. Essentially finite human beings undergo corruption and dissolution. Material finitude expresses itself in such ways as illness, injury, and death.

I suggest that all suffering may be understood as the experience of finitude in tension with intrinsic human dignity. Human beings suffer whenever we become aware of, or experience, our finitude. And finitude is manifested in a myriad of ways. Failure, decay, and mistake are the hallmarks of finitude. Finitude means limitation and imperfection. Particularly in the medical sphere, the fundamental meaning of all loss, injury, illness, pain, and dependence is *death*, the ultimate limit that challenges the notion of human dignity.

Suffering is far wider than physical pain, even in a medical context.[24] Much medical suffering has nothing to do with pain. Suffering may be occasioned by nausea, or dyspnea, or loneliness, or alienation, or rejection. It has been shown, for example, that those who seek euthanasia or physician-assisted suicide usually do so for reasons of suffering other than physical pain.[25]

Just as one can suffer without pain, so one can experience pain without suffering. The pain of putting one's fingers momentarily too close to a flame, for example, hardly counts as suffering. Also, runners and other athletes can experience certain pains as exhilaration, the breaking of some limit; it is only the pain that limits their accomplishments that counts as genuine suffering. Pain hurts, but pain becomes an occasion of suffering because it evokes limitation, altering one's ability to be the person one has been and to do the things one should be able to do. Pain that occasions an experience of limitation points inexorably toward death, and this is why those who are in pain suffer. Suffering is a confrontation with the meaning of finitude. Everything that is called a "material evil" is a material occasion of the experience of the finitude that is essential to the human condition.

Only human beings experience genuine suffering.[26] The pain felt by animals is genuine evil to the extent that the primitive animal consciousness can grasp this as a limit, but the animal can have no grasp of any tension between limitation and dignity. Animals do not have this dignity, nor the capacity for this sort of consciousness. It is an act of anthropomorphic interpretation by which we attribute suffering to animals that are in pain.

The pain of children and the demented is also genuine evil to the extent that it is grasped, however primitively, as limitation. But their pain is suffering only to the extent that these suffering creatures have intrinsic human dignity and that we can interpret their pain and limitation as fundamentally in tension with that dignity. Thus, a person in a persistent vegetative state can still be said to suffer, even in the absence of pain, because the limitations of that state are in tension with the dignity that we believe the patient has as a human person.

An important consequence of this understanding is that it takes a broad metaphysical view of the whole problem of theodicy. The fundamental category is finitude, a category that is wider than Leibniz's "metaphysical evil." Finitude is not just one type of evil alongside two other types, material and moral. Finitude is the fundamental metaphysical category at the heart of the problem of evil, whether material or moral. Finitude is simply a metaphysical truth, in itself neither good nor evil.

Much of the world's finitude is premoral and spatiotemporal—the decay of mu mesons or the erosion of cliffs, for example. These sorts of phenomena are beautiful and interesting parts of the finite, created universe and each, in itself, is good. Some spatiotemporal finitude, however, constitutes material evil inasmuch as it causes human suffering. To the extent that any of these physical phenomena interacts with the physical phenomenon of a human body in such a way as to accelerate or to provoke the finitude of that human body, that phenomenon is, in this sense, evil. A hurricane is not in itself evil. It is an evil if it destroys human shelter, disrupts human communication, or injures human beings—if it is an occasion of human suffering. The malarial parasite is not, in itself, evil. If it affected only mosquitoes no one would worry. It is evil to the extent that it causes human morbidity and mortality: fever, anemia, weakness, or death. In themselves, as created, finite entities, even storms and parasites are good.

Moral finitude, on the other hand, results from imperfections in human beliefs and choices, and may manifest itself as a failure in reason, will, or desire. The moral finitude for which human beings can be found blameworthy is moral evil. Other human beings may be caused to suffer through a person's moral failures either in a direct, interpersonal manner or indirectly through the creation of conditions that cause someone to experience his or her material finitude.

Everything that is created is necessarily finite, including human beings. Whatever apprehends its own finitude as an experience in tension with its intrinsic dignity suffers. It is through the *meaning* of loss, pain, dependence, and death that human beings suffer. These are concrete expressions of human finitude. To be human is to suffer. It could not be otherwise.

Human beings are imperfect, limited, fallible creatures. We are imperfect in our beliefs and choices, and imperfect in our embodied existence. We are limited in our moral life and limited in our embodied days (see Job 14:4–5). Suffering is the experience of these limits.

Types of Suffering

The possible occasions of human suffering are unfortunately plentiful. To assist in this analysis, I propose a classification into four types, based on my definition of suffering and the distinction between moral and material evil.

Type I
Human beings can suffer as a result of our own moral evil without any intervening material occasion; examples include the pangs of conscience, remorse, and guilt. This is the experience of personal moral finitude. A physician may feel guilty about having abandoned a patient and recognize his or her limited individual capacity for good. In penance, we confess our moral finitude as undermining our intrinsic dignity.

Type II
Human beings can suffer as a result of the moral evil of others without any intervening material occasion; examples include experiences of loneliness, hurt, and alienation. This is the experience of the moral finitude of others. If one were a patient, one might feel hurt by the cold and relatively inattentive manner in which one was treated by one's physician. No material wound or blow need serve as an intervening occasion of the suffering; the moral failure of the physician is sufficient cause. One recognizes that the world's love is finite.

Type III
Human beings can suffer as a result of the moral evil of self or of others, mediated through material occasions of suffering. The long and horrible list of examples include self-mutilation, torture, assault, rape, poisoning, murder, war, and willful negligence. These are at once experiences of the moral finitude of others and of the material finitude of one's own person. Records and memories of "experiments" performed on Nazi prisoners provide especially egregious medical examples. More subtly, a physician's greed may lead to excessive use of medical technologies with attendant physical harm to some patients.

Type IV
There are a myriad of material occasions of human suffering that require no moral evil whatsoever—the central problems of medical suffering. Examples include fractured bones that result from landslides, inherited diseases like cystic fibrosis and hemophilia, and the relentless commonplaces such as arthritis, dia-

betes, cancer, heart attacks, and strokes. These are personal experiences of material finitude. From the physician's perspective, they can also represent the
physician's own experience of the finitude of medicine. Medicine does not grant
immortality.

Mixed Types

Certainly there can be occasions of suffering that are, in part, directly material
and, in part, the result of moral evil. Multiple combinations and permutations
are possible. Examples could include a person with lung cancer who had a genetic predisposition but who also started smoking at an early age, in part because
greedy tobacco company executives, motivated by a desire for profits, deliberately repressed evidence about the addictive nature of cigarettes and authorized
an advertising campaign aimed at teenagers. The bad genes are a contributing
factor, but the teenager's decision to smoke and the business practices of the
tobacco company played significant roles also.

These categories seem to me more useful than the simple classical division
between moral and material evil. The picture is much more complex than that.

Human Suffering and the Power of God

It might be objected that while I may have found a way to begin to defend the
rationality of believing in God in the face of the reality of human suffering, I
have paid too high a price to do so. One could argue that I have reconciled the
apparent contradiction between belief in an all-powerful, all-loving God and the
existence of evil by denying God's omnipotence. That is, the God I am sketching
seems incapable of creating human beings who could not suffer, and so is not
truly all-powerful.

I respond that this objection rests upon faulty logic. The argument asks, in
effect, whether God, the ground of all reason as well as all love, can be involved
in self-contradiction. But, if all creatures are finite and suffering is the experience
of finitude, then this question is itself internally contradictory. It asks whether
God can make a free, conscious creature that is not a creature; the question
makes no sense. God's power is not diminished by the fact that God cannot
violate the logic God has already ordained.[27]

Material Occasions of Suffering and Human Finitude

Plantinga's free-will defense was designed to show that belief in God is compatible with the existence of moral evil in all its forms. I have objected that his

reduction of all material evil to moral evil solves the logical problem but requires believers to accept a teaching that is not dogmatically necessary, and I suggested instead that the evil that results from material occasions of human suffering may be justified by a metaphysical argument. I have argued that it is the human experience of the material finitude of human existence that constitutes the suffering occasioned by all instances of medical evil that are material in nature.

It might be objected that even if human beings, as creatures, are necessarily finite, no argument has been advanced to explain why it should be necessary that our finitude have a material expression. Why should it be necessary that we be materially finite—and vulnerable to physical suffering? Could God not have limited the finitude of human beings to moral fallibility? If God is really loving and good, would this not have been a better arrangement?

Quite bluntly, my reply to these objections is to note that they boil down to asking for an explanation of why human beings are not something other than human. They ascribe to *Homo sapiens* a possible suprahuman existence. But, "For it is clear that he did not come to help angels, but the descendants of Abraham" (Hebrews 2:16). Our finitude must be *human* finitude. It is the nature of human beings to be material—embodied persons. If human beings had bodies but did not experience death, we would be spirits accidentally inhabiting bodies, not essentially embodied creatures. But we are not pure spirits. To be human, we must be finite in the whole of our existence. Therefore, human beings must be capable of good and evil in our material existence, as well as in our intellectual and moral existence.

This position is decidedly anti-Gnostic. It requires a nonfundamentalist reading of Genesis to accept that human beings are essentially materially finite and that there has never been a historical time without human suffering and death. Current understanding of the biological evolution of human beings raises the question of whether Eden could represent an actual time and place in human history. For many theologians, Eden is now understood to be an expression of the potential with which God endowed human beings—a potential not necessarily ever realized in concrete human history.[28] The basic dogmatic lessons from the Genesis account of creation include the beliefs that God created human beings in the image and likeness of God; that human beings are essentially finite, morally and corporeally; and that God had (or has) other plans for humankind. The compatibility of belief in human evolution and the account of Genesis has been reaffirmed as dogmatically permissible by Pope John Paul II.[29] So it does not seem that the account of human beings as essentially corporeally finite, at least within the history of humankind to which we have access, poses any conceptual or dogmatic problems.

Why So Many Physical Occasions of Suffering?

Physicians, perhaps more than most people, are aware of the extraordinary variety of physical occasions of suffering. Textbooks of medicine and surgery are lengthy catalogs of these horrors: infantile diarrhea, diabetes, cancer, traumatic brain injuries, dementia, and countless other conditions. It might rightly be asked, then, even granting that human beings should be materially finite, why God should allow such a wide variety of ways in which that finitude can be experienced? Could an all-powerful, all-loving, and all-good God not simply have created human beings incapable of experiencing any physical suffering, and have ordained painless sudden death for each person on his or her eighty-fifth birthday? Would such a world not be better than the one we now inhabit? These are significant questions. That human beings, as creatures, must be finite is clear. That human finitude should be expressed in such a variety of ways is not so obvious.

On closer examination, Plantinga's free-will defense of moral evil and my metaphysical defense of physical suffering are not merely parallel arguments. The complete story requires an understanding of the relationship between the two arguments. As Plantinga claims, because freedom is part of what is best about human beings, the best possible kind of human being God could make would be the maximally free human. Therefore, for God's human creatures to be optimal embodied persons, we must be free with respect to our entire essence, not just part of it. As I have argued, because human beings are material creatures, our freedom must pervade all aspects of our material existence. Because human freedom expresses itself in the embodied world in which human beings are active, a world that admits of the greatest possible freedom for moral good expressed through the physical world will also admit of the greatest possible freedom for moral evil expressed through the physical world. Plantinga argues, soundly, that a world with such freedom is better than one that precludes it. This freedom allows human beings to be cocreative with God in forging moral goodness in the physical universe. Unfortunately, it also allows us to unleash Type III suffering into the world.

To have the fullest possible scope of truly significant moral freedom with respect to the world, the necessary concomitant is that there be correlative possibilities for effecting moral evil through manipulation of the material universe. So, for example, the freedom to acquire knowledge about the movement of rivers and about the effects of drought on human populations has resulted in great human accomplishments—the creation of reservoirs, systems of irrigation, and other material occasions of human good. But this same knowledge was used by Machiavelli and Leonardo DaVinci to plan to divert the water supply of an enemy Italian city-state. The freedom to discover that *Bacillus anthracis* is the cause of anthrax has made possible its treatment and cure, and, at the same time, this knowledge has made possible the use of these bacteria in germ warfare. Every significant advance human freedom has creatively wrought in the material universe has brought with it the possibility of some material occasion of human suffering—either by our freely omitting some deed that could bring about a new material good or by our freely choosing to use that advance to create a new occasion of human suffering.

Adopting an argument from Plantinga, I argue that for God to limit any potential for human beings to manipulate the world, for good or for ill, would mean that human beings had been placed in a toy world. Imagine, for instance, that God were to disallow all physical occasions of suffering and arrange for painless sudden death at age eighty-five. This would severely restrict human freedom. We would not be free to choose materially to benefit each other, because we would have no material wants; no acts of charity would be possible. Indeed, not even murder would be possible because we would not be free to choose to kill (or not to kill) any human being. This would hardly constitute maximal human freedom.

Hick has offered a series of thought experiments that supplement this argument based on maximal freedom.[30] He argues that a world without any physical occasions of suffering would be a very odd one. There could be no corporal works of mercy. There would be no Albert Schweitzers and no Mother Teresas because no one would need their services. There would be no medical or nursing professions because there could be no sickness. There would be no courage, because there could be no such thing as danger or a person in need of rescue.

Swinburne makes an important contribution to this line of argument by pointing out that the knowledge necessary to have maximal significant moral freedom with respect to the material world comes only through human experience.[31] For us to be free to refrain from murder, there must have been a first instance in which a material occasion of human suffering occurred from which a human being made the inductive inference that he or she could freely replicate that event. Perhaps someone, somewhere, sometime long ago, saw a rock from a landslide hit another person in the head and cause death. From that experience, the observer learned both a way to murder and a way to protect fellow human beings. But if that particular material occasion of human suffering had not already existed, neither lesson would have been learned. Thus, Swinburne argues, to maximize human freedom with respect to the material world, it is necessary that the variety of material occasions of good and suffering be very great indeed.

So it does not seem absolutely certain that it would have been better for God to have created a world in which the embodied, physical, material occasions of human suffering were as limited as possible while still consistent with the finitude necessary to the concept of creatureliness and to the freedom that is God's great gift to us. It is at least possible, if not probable, that God could not create finite beings who are embodied, thinking, significantly free with respect to moral choices, and as good as they could be given those conditions, without also making possible a multiplicity of material occasions of human suffering.

Suffering and Justice

Others might argue that a mere defense of the compatibility of belief in God, given the volume and variety of evil in the world, is not enough. The protest often is not that God ought not to allow suffering at all, but rather that God ought not to be so unjust in the distribution of suffering. This is a common complaint in the psalms. Contemporary versions are familiar: Why should my cousin, who is so good, suffer from leukemia, while that scoundrel of a landlord, who continuously overcharges poor people and regularly uses women as objects of sexual gratification, is rolling in cash and healthy as a horse? Why do those who are morally evil seem to be relatively free of material suffering, while those who are morally good seem to suffer more?

Whether this is an empirically truthful observation probably cannot be verified. In truth, I suspect that the amount of suffering in the world is rather randomly distributed. The shapes and varieties differ. The relative proportions of material and moral suffering, the times and places in which suffering occurs, the types of suffering differ. But there are no units of suffering. The varieties are incommensurable, and quantitative comparison is not possible. Yet everyone must suffer, for this is the human condition. And one cannot escape from suffering by being either good or bad.

Further, as Donald Nicholl has observed, if everything always and everywhere were to go right for us, and we were never to experience failure or suffering, each of us would quickly become a monster.[32] Through our own experience of finitude, compassion for those who have *their* own personal experiences of finitude becomes easier.

Suffering and Pain

Still, it might be objected that God need not have used pain as the signal to human beings that we are finite. All I have argued thus far is that human beings suffer if we apprehend our finitude. Is it not enough that a patient lose a limb to diabetes? That patient certainly apprehends his or her finitude thereby. Why must it also *hurt*? Worse still, why should that patient also experience the medical phenomenon of *phantom* pain, so that the pain continues as if the gangrenous limb were still there even after it has been amputated?

The standard response to this sort of question has been a defense of the biological utility of pain. Pain is a strong signal; it demands attention. It saves life and limb. For instance, if a child should place his or her hand in a fire, the child feels pain, removes the limb before losing it to the flames, and learns to avoid such dangers in the future. So, the argument goes, pain does more good than harm in the long run.

I find this argument unsatisfactory, particularly as a general internist. Such an argument might have some immediate plausibility with respect to acute pain, but it has no plausibility whatsoever with respect to chronic pain. Chronic pain, like many other chronic conditions that I treat, is a biological adaptation which, while acutely useful for survival, in the long term causes problems of its own. For example, in congestive heart failure the chronic hyperadrenergic state that accompanies this condition is helpful initially in insuring survival but, in the long haul, is maladaptive and destructive or purposeless. The same may be said of chronic pain. There is no biological survival advantage to chronic pain. It seems to serve no purpose; it seems to do more harm than good.

The only reasonable argument, although not an explanation, I can offer is that pain itself, even as a signaling system, is subject to and expressive of the finitude of the human. Pain is not a perfect signaling system. It functions well at times, but its function is limited. With chronicity, pain becomes counterproductive. Pain has a biological purpose but does not achieve that biological purpose perfectly. Human beings are imperfect morally, imperfect intellectually, and imperfect neurologically. Pain is the imperfect warning system we have been given. We cannot explain why we have this particular system, but at least we can know that a hypothetically perfect system would be incompatible with our condition as creatures.

The Limits of Logic and Metaphysics

What I have offered is a defense of the compatibility of belief in God and the existence of medical suffering. I have not offered an explanation of evil. I have only tried to show that what begins as a question about an apparent logical contradiction turns out not to be a question of logic after all. The question raised by suffering in the medical setting is about the meaning of the human condition. To be human is to be a finite creature. As conscious, reflective, free, and finite creatures, we must inevitably experience our own finitude. The experiences of finitude that occur through illness, injury, and death are the physical occasions of medical suffering. To question why we suffer is to raise the question of who and what we are as creatures.

Human beings fail—in love, marriage, child-rearing, and career. We become sick; we die. We are creatures, not gods. This is a fact. It cannot be otherwise. It cannot be further explained. But it also cannot be said that a creature's self-affirmation of creaturehood contradicts that creature's affirmation of a Creator. Logic and metaphysics can say little more.

For the Christian, then, the issue of suffering, understood as the experience of finitude, raises questions about the meaning of human existence and the relationship between God and humankind. Suffering also raises Christological questions. One must grapple with the meaning of the Incarnation, in which the infinite God took on the finitude of the human condition. One must confront the meaning of the suffering of Christ and attempt to understand the claim that this suffering is redemptive.

Suffering Cannot Be Eliminated, Only Transcended

Suffering can be alleviated, but it cannot be completely eliminated. In the end, it can only be transcended. It is impossible to be human and not to suffer. One can escape suffering only if one is not a creature. To suffer is to experience finitude. The fundamental fact of our finite status as creatures is death, the ultimate experience of the finitude that each of us suffers.

This does not imply that we have no duty to try to remove the material occasions of human suffering. On the contrary, Christian charity demands that we do so. Compassion and respect for the dignity of the one who suffers require time, attention, conversation, touching, pain control, and care. But, to eradicate suffering altogether would entail the eradication of the humanity of the sufferer, and respect for persons requires nothing less than absolute respect for their humanity.

Christian faith affirms that only in love can suffering be transcended. Only love has the infinite character that points beyond the finitude of the human condition. Compassion reaches beyond the pain, alienation, loneliness, and despair of those who suffer illness and injury. In compassion, one can use human freedom to remove the material occasions of suffering and overcome the interpersonal barriers that divide us from each other and from God.

Christians believe that through his life, death, and resurrection, Jesus Christ has pointed out the way of transcendence, beyond the horizon of human finitude into the infinity of God. Each Christian must search for meaning in his or her own life in relation to the life of Christ, who has entered into human history and has called each one by name. This call occurs both in caring for the patient who is suffering and in experiencing one's own suffering as a patient. The problem of suffering and faith is not a logical problem, but an invitation to enter into a relationship with God. This is why I so often feel that I must take off my shoes before I enter the room of a patient who is dying in faith, hope, and love. Face to face with the finitude of death, all the reality of human suffering and all the possibilities for transcendence can become clear. The love of God calls us forth from our finitude. The space around a patient who has engaged these questions seriously is holy ground. The horizon is present, and I stand in awe when I see it unfold as something that is not denied but transcended. The One Who Is calls out from the passionate flames. Logic has brought us to the edge of Mystery. It can bring others to that Mystery as well.

7

The Practice of Theodicy

Wendy Farley

Theodicy is usually understood as an intellectual practice that attempts to justify the presence of evil in a world presumably created by a good and all-powerful God. It is often conceived of as a logical conundrum, wherein three mutually exclusive terms are jury-rigged into compatibility.[1] Even supposing one is very clever about reducing the tension among evil, power, and goodness, it is not clear to me that this exercise is particularly useful to anyone actually encountering suffering. Suffering yearns more for experiences of healing presence than for logical arguments. Theory can provide some meaning to suffering, but it is in compassionate relationship that suffering discovers redemption.

Theodicy moves from irrelevance to something closer akin to evil itself when its job is envisioned to be the development of theories that judge experienced suffering as nonevil.[2] Much, though certainly not all, of classical Christian theology is dedicated to showing that suffering is not unjust. A common way of doing this is to argue that suffering coincides with just desert. The universality of guilt means that no suffering could in principle exceed what people deserve to suffer. Conversely, it becomes axiomatic that if there is suffering there must be guilt; fault is inferred simply from the fact of suffering itself.

Richard Zaner gives an example of this theodicy in action in a story of a two-year-old boy born with "short-gut" syndrome. The boy's parents were children of fundamentalists, and the pregnancy occurred prior to their marriage. "When the baby was born and its problems known, the parents were informed that this was 'God's punishment' for their sins." Largely because of this theological interpretation of their situation, they became somewhat withdrawn from their beloved son.

> Little wonder, we all thought when this story became known, that these young people had been acting oddly. They had to contend with their child's condition and continuous hospitalization, their own sense of having possibly done something to make it happen, and then the constant accusations from both families that they had indeed been sinful and made to suffer God's wrath.[3]

The way we interpret suffering has a great deal to do with how we experience suffering. The intensification of the suffering of this couple by the use of religion to claim that they and their child deserved to suffer is an unfortunate exemplification of theodicy as itself an evil.[4]

Yet, amid the assaults of suffering, the survival of meaningfulness is intrinsic to the resistance of suffering. When theodicy contributes to this struggle for meaning, it becomes part of a practice that resists evil. Theodicy can best do this by dispensing with the standard formulation of the problem of evil: If God is all-powerful and perfectly good, why is there evil in the world? This question throws up a steep barricade of theory against the immediacy of the pain that provokes the question in the first place. It also imports the uncriticized presupposition that the nature of God's power is as absolute causation. Many theologians have been willing to accept any suffering as God's will rather than discard the belief that God causes and wills everything that human beings experience. But, as I shall suggest in a later section, there is much in scripture itself, as well as in experience and the theological tradition, to challenge this assertion.

As a practice that is both a meaningful interpretation of suffering and a response to suffering, theodicy must avoid alienating abstractions as well as oppressive images of God. Instead of beginning with a logical conundrum, we must begin with the understanding that theodicy's initial subject matter is raw pain. Sometimes pain is temporary, agonizing in the moment, but giving way to future healing. But sometimes pain does not open onto healing. It is the pain of permanent loss, loss of health or capacity or life or love. Theodicy's proper subject matter is the shock of permanent loss: the face that has been burned off, the beloved child whose beautiful little soul has flickered out, the discovery of an illness that promises to strip away one's mind before finally surrendering the body to death. Human capacities for understanding and compassion are radically undermined when we school ourselves in indifference to suffering's power. The proper work of theodicy is to help purge us of this temptation. In place of an immediate effort to professionalize, rationalize, or justify suffering, we must first contemplate suffering, just as the medieval mystics contemplated the wounds of Christ. If we allow ourselves to draw near to the facticity of suffering, we may be less tempted to allow a theoretical construct (whether theological or professional) to stand in for the painfulness of human experience.

Theodicy is a justification, that is, a "making right" of evil. Leibniz coined the term to express the way philosophy and theology attempt to justify God's goodness in light of evil. But suffering is not made right in a theory. If suffering can be justified at all it is in action and relationship, in the actual events of human life. Reflection on suffering may contribute a little life raft of meaning when the seas are rough. If sufferers and those who care for them inhabit a conceptual world in which dignity can be maintained when body and soul are under assault, the dehumanizing intensity of suffering can be challenged. Just as the merciless theodicy Zaner describes in the story of the child dying of short-gut syndrome can work much mischief, so maintaining the belief and experience of God's goodness in the midst of suffering can contribute to the courage to endure. But justification does not occur primarily in ideas. It is manifest in the fullest sense only in the enactment of an alternative to the degradations suffering inflicts. If we understand theodicy to be not merely an intellectual exercise but a justification, a making right, of suffering, then we are invited to interpret theodicy as a practice of compassion. There is no theory that makes it "okay" for children to be racked by the pain of long disease, or for older people to be defrauded of their life stories by dementia, or for parents to be taken from their children by random cancer. If life is meaningful and good even though it is fraught on all sides with these possibilities—and always also with the intransigence of death— it is because some other reality is lived out *all the time*. It is because life is laced with the practices of compassion that pain and death are deprived of the final word.

In the next section I shall identify difficulties that can make the loving presence of God in the midst of suffering unintelligible. Theodicy cannot provide the correct answer to why people suffer. But it can go ever more deeply into the compassionate womb of God by stripping away lies about who God is and who we are. Theory begins and ends in practices. In the following section, I shall describe theodicy as a practice, and one that is of critical importance to those whose profession places them in relation to people at the extremity of the human condition.

"And I Saw No Wrath Anywhere"

Being in labor for a birth of a child nails one to the nonnegotiable reality of embodied existence. It does not matter how one prepared, whether one desired to get pregnant, what one believes, or what kind of person one is—the body will take its own course and a woman must ride that wave wherever it takes her. It is like (and perhaps *is*) being plunged into the throbbing center of the ocean where life and death were first formed. The power of that place makes human willing seem very small indeed because it overwhelms our desires and appears utterly indifferent to them. If all goes well, labor calls forth a baby, pinched and beautiful, and opens one more deeply to the adventure of life.

Suffering has something of this intransigent character. It is utterly indifferent to us as persons and can overwhelm us entirely. In a different context, Elaine Scarry reminds us of the way pain displaces us more radically than anything else can:

It is a commonplace that at the moment when a dentist's drill hits and holds an exposed nerve, a person sees stars. What is meant by "seeing stars" is that the contents of consciousness are, during those moments, obliterated, that the name of one's child, the memory of a friend's face, are all absent.[5]

There is something about the assault on the body that tears meaning to pieces. As doctors have reason to know, we are, in a certain sense, our bodies. We do not exist independently from them, wearing our bodies indifferently like cloaks that have nothing to do with us. We all know we will die but when we are faced with our own death or the death of a child or other loved one, that knowledge is transformed from general, abstract information into the unmaking of the world. How can the world be good, how can there be a God, if such a thing can happen to my little child, to my body, to *me*? These are not logical questions; they are pleas for redemptive power.

The possibility of experiencing redemptive power can be blocked when we forget who we are and forget the essential goodness of God. This existential forgetfulness can help suffering gain dominion over us. We can forget we have bodies, forget that we die, and instead expect that we should live somewhat like characters in situation comedies or models in toothpaste ads who seem both untouched and untouchable by physical diminishment. This point must be made carefully. By calling attention to our physical vulnerability and our mortality, I do not mean that sickness and pain should not be resisted or that healing should not be sought. But our culture has become so preoccupied with the apparently infinite possibilities for healing and with a kind of horror at any kind of physical imperfection that we have few categories for thinking theologically and ethically about our *nature* as embodied and therefore mortal beings.[6] A hatred or denial of the conditions of life does little to prepare us for the inevitable sufferings every human being encounters. The Christian tradition, for all its reservations about bodies, does understand the distinctively human form of existence (spiritual, rational beings with bodies, embedded in a natural world) as good and beautiful, created deliberately by God for God's and our own delight.[7] The theological idea of createdness need not be interpreted mythologically but rather as a claim that the human condition, fraught as it is with suffering, has a kind of beauty and dignity to it. If we understand that suffering is inevitable and death the signature of the kind of being we are, these things may come less as meaningless assaults. Underneath the raw pain of loss, there might remain a deep sense of the integrity of our being and the presence of God with us in ways that accord with our nature.

We cannot remain deceived about our nature and expect to endure gracefully the sufferings to which we are subject. Yet it is equally a part of our nature to experience suffering and death as in some sense alien to us, as Tolstoy demonstrates in his story about Ivan Ilych's dying:

In the depth of his heart he knew he was dying, but not only was he not accustomed to the thought, he simply did not and could not grasp it.

The syllogism he had learnt from Kiezewetter's Logic "Caius is a man, men are mortal, therefore Caius is mortal," had always seemed to him correct as applied to Caius, but certainly not as applied to himself. That Caius—man in the abstract— was mortal, was perfectly correct, but he was not Caius, not an abstract man, but a creature quite, quite separate from all others. He had been little Vanya, with a mamma and a papa. . . . "Caius really was mortal and it was right for him to die; but for me, little Vanya, Ivan Ilych, with all my thoughts and emotions, it's altogether a different matter. It cannot be that I ought to die. That would be too terrible."[8]

Human beings seem made for life, not death. In our thirst for happiness and life, there is no hint that we are made for death and suffering; these come to us as strangers and enemies. As Ivan continues: "If I had to die like Caius I should have known it was so. An inner voice would have told me so, but there was nothing of the sort in me and I and all my friends felt that our case was quite different from that of Caius." Tolstoy describes here the paradoxical character of the existential encounter with death. What we know to be completely universal nonetheless approaches us individually as a shock and affront.

Classical Christian theology describes the evil of death and suffering as a privation of being.[9] My students, upon hearing this, are immediately skeptical and dissatisfied; they believe it is a "weak" sense of evil. But it means that we are defrauded of something not only proper to us, but essential to our very being. To be deprived of sight or health or life itself is not like being deprived of a new bike. It is a deprivation of some good that is constitutive of our very being. This deprivation, this defrauding, of the kind of existence we are intended for is what Christian theologians have meant by "natural evil." It is because physical pain, loss, and death are privations of our very being that they always come to us contingently and, somehow, unfairly. The interpretation of natural suffering as privation points to a deep paradox in our nature. We are mortal, yet experience our mortality as entirely improper to us. We, like Ivan Ilych, know that all people are mortal. But the death of our children, the anguish of long illness, the discovery that our parents are failing all come as violations.

It is our nature to have an unbearably paradoxical nature: to be mortal and yet to experience this mortality as contingent, a surprise, an injustice. Biblical symbols articulate this paradox: We are dust and to dust we will return (Genesis 3:19). And yet we are also made in the image of God (Genesis 1:27). We are these strange creatures made of dust and the divine image (or as Buddhists put it, we all possess the Buddha mind). There is something endlessly beautiful about us, perfectly good, shining and bright as the sun. It is this image of God in us that suffering defaces. Suffering and death tell us that we are nothing but our bodies; they pin us to our bodies and insist we have no other dignity or loveliness. When my friend was dying of leukemia, very soon before his death he suffered terrible diarrhea. At one point he cried out in despair, "I have nothing left but shit to give to God." This is one of the lies impressed upon us by suffering. Succumbing to the lie (which he did not) that we are nothing, that we are shit, that we lack the golden image of God woven indelibly into our souls, grants to suffering almost complete power over us.

One useful work theodicy can perform is to remind us who we are: not only that we are mortal but that we are persons of great beauty and dignity. We are human beings and this means that we are embodied, but embodied beings with spirits. We are bodies that possess the untarnished image of God. Roberta Bondi, the fine patristics scholar, provided a contemporary reflection on the meaning of the theological notion of the image of God within us in an analysis of the Lord's Prayer:

> "Hallowed be your name," I said next, and as I said it I recalled again my teacher Cyprian, who had reminded his third-century congregation in Carthage that because God's name is already holy, what Jesus must have intended us to ask for here was that God's name be made holy in us.[10]

My friend with leukemia gave a powerful testimony to the difficulty and beauty of this lesson: God's image can be made holy in us in the midst of the humiliations and pain our bodies suffer. This reflection is very important for "medical" or "natural" suffering. Theodicy reminds us not to despise suffering or ourselves as sufferers. It reminds us that it is as embodied beings, subject to the horrors of embodied existence, that the distinctively human image of God appears in us. God is mirrored in us not *despite* our bodies but precisely *because* we are the kind of spiritual beings that have this kind of body.[11] This does not mean that the body's suffering does not cause the deepest anguish. It does not mean that facile words to a "body in pain" about the image of God will ameliorate suffering one iota. It does mean that suffering does not erode our most basic beauty as possessors of God's image. Theodicy requires us to deepen our capacity to see this beauty in ourselves and in all others and to respond to others in light of this beauty, however racked and defaced by pain it may be. Suffering evokes horror in those who observe it and humiliation in those who suffer it. But the practice of theodicy reminds us of the real being of the sufferer and invites us to act according to the soul's beauty rather than be distracted by the ugliness of suffering.

Somehow we must constantly school ourselves in ever deeper awareness of these two dimensions of our nature: our mortality and our beauty. We must understand that suffering and death are privations of our nature *and* that it is our nature to be vulnerable to these privations. The fruit of this knowledge should be an increasingly genuine and profound compassion for the kind of being we are, torn between these two realities.

Observing and experiencing suffering can contribute to misunderstandings of our nature. They can also contribute to unhelpful interpretations of divine power. An important task of theodicy is to undermine the temptation to conceive of suffering as a form of divine punishment. Because the body is a condition of human existence, and the body is subject to pain, and God is in some sense the ground or creator of our being, it is possible, in this inferential sense, to say that God "wills" suffering.[12] This means only that the condition of our existence is tragically structured, that its good is contingent upon vulnerability to evil. But to say that God desires (if this anthropomorphism can be used) our existence and its conditions is not the same as saying that God in some direct way wills each particular suffering in and for itself. Roberta Bondi attributes the accompaniment of suffering by the experience of guilt as a sign of alienation from God that God's presence helps assuage:

> "Your will be done" were the next words of my prayer. "My God," I prayed, "I know that when I am demoralized and full of panic and grief, I am tempted to believe that my pain is somehow your will, your desired punishment for my failures. I really do know how gently you regard all our wounds, all the things that hurt us. . . . Our God, because I can't seem to retain it for myself, I need you to remind me constantly that what you desire for all people, including for me and for little Roberta, is our well-being and our health."[13]

Theodicy invites us to reflect on the meaning of suffering in light of some idea of who God is and how God is related to the world. The most basic clue we have about who God is is the experience of redemption. In the Hebrew Scriptures this is talked about first as the miracle of creation itself and then as the liberation of slaves from the empire of Egypt. It is the founding of a community upon principles of justice and dedication to God. The Christian Scriptures describe the inbreaking of ultimate reality as a *metanoia*: a turning around and upside down of persons and societies that enables one to participate with heart and body, soul and mind and community in the living reality of love and compassion. The Christian Scriptures end with a vibrantly colorful vision of a time when the ultimate reality of compassionate power becomes transparent to history, in some definitive way overcoming evil. The Buddhist tradition likewise understands awakening to ultimate reality as generative of *mahakaruna*, great compassion. In this tradition, the awakened one embodies compassion that is perfectly universal and that is quickened by the desire and power to liberate others from suffering. In both of these traditions, compassion is the fundamental signature of ultimate reality.

Religious traditions are anything but unanimous about the interpretation of their scriptures, but these indications about the effects of divine power provide important clues for developing an understanding of who God is and how God is related to suffering. Suffering can cause human beings to despise themselves and one another. This is often projected onto God, as if God delighted in human suffering. But the presence of divine power in experiences of redemption points in an entirely different direction. Divine power is the empowering of beauty, life, love. Christian Neoplatonists understand God as the Good beyond being, itself beyond every category of thought or being but the source of all that is and, therefore, the power that generates each thing in its distinctive beauty and joy.[14] To be good is the nature of God, not an arbitrary decision God makes one day and reneges on the next. God *is* good. The Christian narrative reinforces this claim. The most basic beginning point of the narrative is the incarnation, the embodiment of ultimate truth in a cowshed. The penultimate conclusion is the crucifixion, in which Christ enters into human suffering and despair as radically as possible. In this radical presencing, God is with us precisely in our mortality. God does not so much explain evil as respond to it. "And the Word became flesh and lived among us" (John 1:14). God will "wipe away every tear from their eyes. Death will be no more; mourning and crying and pain will be no more" (Revelation 21:4). The incarnation, the crucifixion, and eschatological hopes are not theses to be believed or not, but signatures of the way in which God relates to suffering. The Christian mystical tradition also reinforces this knowledge of the imperturbable goodness of God: "For I saw most truly that where our Lord appears, peace is received and wrath has no place; for I saw no kind of wrath in God, neither briefly nor for long . . . For though we may feel in ourselves anger, contention and strife, still we are all mercifully enclosed in God's mildness and . . . meekness, in [God's] benignity and . . . accessibility."[15]

We discover God not in what tears us apart but in what enables us to endure. The power of God is most distinctively evident in the power of life and beauty. This means that we must learn where to seek God in the midst of suffering. In our misery, we can sometimes imagine God as the agent of misery. We think of God as having a kind of power that totalitarian governments fantasize for themselves: a power that utterly and perfectly controls not only every event but even the interior workings of the human soul. Some parents lust after this sort of power to control their children's minds, actions, hearts. Such parents and governments inflict humiliating sufferings in order to destroy in people whatever does not coincide with their will. The exercise of this kind of power, however imperfect, is invariably destructive. It reduces beautiful human souls to rags of suffering and ethical paralysis. To imagine that the kind of power that is most destructive of us is the kind of power that animates the universe seems both immoral and theologically inconsistent. When this cruelly omnipotent deity is understood to be the only theological option, a rejection of religion in any form can seem a necessary response. One is left with only two deeply destructive alternatives: to embrace a troubling image of God or reject God altogether.

The practice of theodicy should help purge us of these twin toxins. We do not have to project onto God ideas of power that are harmful and immoral. Rather, we must explore how God, if God is truly good, is present to us even when we suffer. H. Richard Niebuhr, the great twentieth-century ethicist, has written: "Responsibility affirms: 'God is acting in all actions upon you. So respond to all actions upon you as to respond to his [sic] action.'"[16] This is a dangerous statement because it is so close to being right. The radical intensity of God's presence to the world is the essential content of the Christian gospel. Paul describes a radical power of God that makes us "more than conquerors" in the midst of affliction (Romans 8:37). He writes of the ineffaceable presence of God amid terrible trials. "For I am convinced that neither death, nor life, nor angels, nor rulers, nor things present, nor things to come, nor powers, nor height, nor depth, nor anything else in all creation, will be able to separate us from the love of God" (Romans 8:38–39). Niebuhr is representative of much theology—whether conservative, liberal, or neo-orthodox—that insists God is acting upon us in what we suffer, that is, creating the conditions of our suffering. This would require that we understand every action upon us—cancer, neonatal intensive care units, burns, kidney failure, AIDS—as God's action upon us. If we believe this, we must torture ourselves to submit not only to the diminishment caused by affliction but to an excruciating alienation from God. But Paul does not say that God causes our afflictions. He says rather that nothing that the world can throw at us—tortures, hunger, persecution—removes God's love from us. Love is not a sentimental feeling; it is a power, a power that is not mastered by anything that happens to us. We should not look for divine power in the events that rip us to shreds. We must learn to look for God as the power that holds us together even when we are being ripped to shreds. When our bodies are dismembered by sickness or accident, there may be nothing but pure pain for a while. But God is burning in us as our beauty that is not dismembered, as love for us that is pure and undiluted, as whatever power we have to endure what must be endured and to surrender when surrender is proper.

When we suffer and when we are in the presence of suffering, it is especially easy to forget the luster of goodness that is at the heart of the human being and it is easy to forget, if we ever knew, the unquenchable goodness of divine power. It is therefore the most important work of theodicy to insist always and with as much passion, intelligence, and skillful means as can be mustered that God is good. "For this is the property of God which opposes good to evil. So Jesus Christ, who opposes good to evil, is our true Mother. We have our being from him, where the foundation of motherhood begins, with all the sweet protection of love which endlessly follows."[17] God is good not in spite of the fact that "he" tortures us. God is good because God is compassionate to us in our pain, loving in our indignities, a constant presence—even if unknown, unfelt—in our despair

and absence from ourselves. God is the power through which our bones are knitted and reknitted together; God is the power through which our soul shines with
a silver luster. When our bodies are unmade and our souls defaced, God abides
with us. God loves the kind of being we are; God is not disgusted by our fragilities
but loves who we are. We are mortal and, therefore, subject to pain, loss, and
death. This is the kind of being we are; these characteristics are not each a special work of God. It is the distinctive power of God to redeem this kind of being
and therefore bring redemptive power to the places of suffering and despair. The
work of theodicy that accompanies us all our lives, as sufferers and companions
to sufferers, is to find and keep an immediate awareness of the ultimate truth
which is the heart of religion and yet constantly displaced by religion: God is
good.

De Profundis

> Out of the depths I cry to you, O Lord. Lord, hear my voice! Let your ears be
> attentive to the voice of my supplications! . . . I wait for the Lord, my soul waits,
> and in his word I hope; my soul waits for the Lord more than those who watch for
> the morning. (Psalm 130:1–2, 5–6)

If suffering were to be made intelligible, that might help us retain, at various
times in our lives, an experience of meaningfulness in the face of our own and
others' suffering. But suffering does not require explanation so much as redemption. There simply do not exist words or ideas or concepts that can undo the
savagery of the suffering to which we are subject as creatures with bodies and
loved ones. But what concepts cannot do, relationships can. How human beings
act toward one another has a great deal to do with whether or not we find hope
or grace in the midst of suffering.

I was struck reading Richard Zaner's book, *Troubled Voices*, how little communication occurred between doctors and patients. He tells the story of a toddler
dying of "short-gut" syndrome, mentioned earlier in this chapter. The child had
lived in the hospital for his entire two and a half years of life. At the point when
Zaner came into the story, the boy was very close to the end of what medical care
could accomplish for him; he could no longer take in nutrition. The question for
the team who cared for him, however, was where he was to die. The parents had
not been around much and the doctors had not even met them. At Zaner's suggestion, the parents were contacted and, in the course of conversations between
them and their son's caregivers, it became clear that they desperately wanted to
have their son with them and to care for him themselves as he died. After a few
months, the child died "peacefully in their arms. A letter from the couple expressed their deep gratitude for having been enabled to express themselves and

have time with their son." Discussions that enabled humane decisions to be made about the child and his parents occurred because of the presence of this "professional" ethicist on the staff at Vanderbilt's hospital. He did not give them any particular advice, but simply became "a trigger for very crucial conversations."[18] These conversations, which "had not been thought appropriate" by many on the team, are the essential stuff of theodicy: They are the place where evil is encountered and resisted.

Why should this or any child be born without the capacity to take in nutrition? No human being can answer that question and those who insist they know should be viewed with some suspicion. We cannot explain away suffering. But it is possible to be present to one another in our suffering. "People who are sick or injured not only want to know what's wrong, why they're hurting, what can be expected . . . but also want to know whether anybody *cares*, whether the people who take care *of* them also care *for* them."[19] Human suffering is the suffering of beings of infinite worth; in the face of suffering their bodies need attention, but their sense of dignity is perhaps even more integral to them. It is not medical technology but relationships that mediate dignity to each of us.

> To come across this phenomenon of *worth* is to learn something very significant about ourselves. We *are enabled to be* what we are only within these complex and mutual relationships with others, relationships which voice that complex and often troubled imperative. We need and want other people to know that each of us is important, and we need and want to know that we matter to them. . . . To be present with the sick or maimed is to find and feel oneself *called on*. Just here, one sees the real significance of plain talk, a simple touch, the direct look . . . that simple human touch, the sound of a human voice, the notice in the human look appear as touchstones of the moral order and enable the person to know in the most immediate way that he or she is recognized and affirmed. This act of affirming of one another, of being with one another in our mutual relatedness, is the hearthstone of our common humanity.[20]

Compassion is the power to taste simultaneously the indignity of affliction and the beauty of the sufferer. This tasting enables one to be present to others so that they can, in turn, feel this indignity and beauty given back to them. Suffering cannot be justified, but it can be transformed when it is blessed by compassion. For this reason, compassion is theodicy's ultimate work. Ideas that try to explain or justify suffering have a place in human culture. But they do not do what suffering most requires: They do not redeem suffering. Compassion sees the ugliness of pain and mirrors back the beauty of the image of God. It does this always according to the concrete requirements of a particular situation, within the always changing needs of individual persons and through the unique beauty compassion takes on as it is embodied in different people.[21] It is not logic but power that resists the ultimacy of evil. It is the perilous gift to the human race that we can be conduits of that power. It does not free us from our wrenching mortality, but it can bring light and a taste of life's beauty to the most desperate places.

In the Christian narrative, God does not explain evil but responds to it, most characteristically by communion with us. This compassionate presencing is the only answer to evil we seem to get. It is this in which we are invited to participate as possessors of the divine image. The power of compassion is the antidote to suffering that assuages its ravages. It is the vocation of every human being that exists, or ever will exist, to penetrate the heart of suffering with this elixir, which cannot change our nature but nonetheless brings a taste of another reality.[22]

Postscript

Because, I suppose, academic chapters are intended to have a neatness to them, a clear beginning, middle, and end, mine has culminated in a proper conclusion. But, this structure is out of keeping with its subject matter. Evil seeks redemption, but it does not always get it. Compassion is an "answer" to evil precisely because there is no answer. If my two-and-a-half-year-old Paul died in my arms, you can be sure I would be tasting not any of life's beauty, but rather pure, unbearable, crushing pain. It is the nature of suffering to deprive us of goods necessary to us and this deprivation can only be searingly painful. Theodicy does not change that. Compassion answers suffering by sitting with it and sharing the knowledge of pain. It is to this communion that we are all elected and it is in this communion that we become friends of God.

8

Rabbi, Why Does God Make Me Suffer?

Elliot N. Dorff

Judaism's positions on issues in health care stem from three of its underlying principles, i.e., that the body belongs to God; that the body is integrated into the entire human person and, as such, is morally neutral, its moral valence being determined by how we use our physical abilities; and that human beings have both the permission and the obligation to heal.

1. *The body belongs to God.* For Judaism, God owns everything, including our bodies.[1] God loans them to us for the duration of our lives, and they are returned to God when we die. The immediate implication of this principle is that neither men nor women have the right to govern their bodies as they will. Because God created our bodies and owns them, God can and does assert the right to restrict the use of our bodies according to the rules articulated in Jewish law.

One set of rules requires us to take reasonable care of our bodies.[2] Another obligates us to avoid danger and injury.[3] Ultimately, human beings do not, according to Judaism, have the right to commit suicide, for that would be a total obliteration of that which belongs to God.[4]

2. *The body is morally neutral and potentially good.* The second major principle underlying Jewish medical ethics is that the body is morally neutral and potentially good. For Judaism the body is as much the creation of God as the mind, the will, and the emotions are. Its energies, like those of our other faculties, are morally neutral, but they can and should be used for divine purposes as defined by Jewish law and tradition.[5] Within that structure, the body's pleasures are God-given and are not to be shunned, for that would be an act of ingratitude toward our Creator.[6] The body, in other words, can and should give us pleasure to the extent that that fits within its overriding purpose of enabling us to live a life of holiness.

The medical implications of this are clear. Jews have the obligation to maintain health not only to care for God's property, but also so that they can accomplish their purpose in life, i.e., to live a life of holiness.

3. *Human beings are not only permitted, but obliged to try to heal.* God's owner-

115

ship of our bodies is also behind our obligation to seek medical help to prevent and cure disease in ourselves and others.[7] Human medical interventions are not construed as acts of human hubris, interfering in what God decreed; on the contrary, we are all under the divine imperative to serve as God's agents and partners in helping God preserve and protect what is God's.[8]

Undergirding this Jewish demand for providing medical care is the Jewish perspective that suffering is not in and of itself redemptive. With the Passion and Resurrection at the center of Christian faith and symbols, Christian theologians often speak of the redemptive character of suffering. That has never been part of the Jewish perspective. On the Day of Atonement (Yom Kippur) and on historical fast days like Tisha B'Av, we are to "afflict our souls" through fasting, sexual abstinence, and other forms of physical self-denial, but in each case the abstinence is restricted to that day and is designed to call attention to the theme of the day; it is not because the pain itself effects atonement or historical memory. Thus if a person's life is medically endangered on Yom Kippur, the law itself not only permits but requires that the abstinence cease and appropriate measures be taken to insure life and health.[9]

Retroactively, when trying to explain how God could be just even though innocent people suffer, the rabbis suggested, among other approaches, that the pain of the innocent may be "afflictions of love" (*yissurim shel ahavah*) designed by God either to teach the person virtues of patience and faith or to punish the person in this life for his or her small number of sins so as to make his or her reward in the next life pure and all the greater,[10] but that doctrine was never used before the fact to justify withholding pain medication from the suffering. On the contrary, the Talmud records that Rabbi Hiyya bar Abba, Rabbi Yohanon, and Rabbi Eleazar all say that neither their sufferings nor the reward promised in the world to come for enduring them are welcome. That is, they would rather live without both the suffering and the anticipated reward.[11] Thus, from its earliest sources, Judaism has both permitted and required us to act as God's agents in bringing healing or, failing that, in reducing pain.

Classical and Modern Jewish Theodicies

Biblical and rabbinic sources on illness are ambivalent about God's role in it. On the one hand, the Torah asserts that if we obey God, God will prevent illness in the first place and heal it if it occurs; conversely, if we disobey God, God will inflict illness as one form of punishment.[12] On the other hand, the biblical book of Job forcefully questions the linkage between Job's sufferings and any misdeeds on his part. Similarly, rabbinic literature records the view that "there is no suffering without iniquity,"[13] but the rabbis were so distressed by the fact that the good suffer and the evil prosper that they affirmed belief in resurrection after death, when the good would get their due reward and the evil their punishment. Moreover, they vigorously engaged in medical research, despite the presumptive link between sickness and sin, and suggesting that sin was the cause of a person's disease was a forbidden act of verbal oppression.[14] Thus the upshot of classical Jewish sources is that, on the one hand, we would expect a just and good God to inflict illness only on the sinful, but in reality that does not happen.

This is one manifestation of what theologians call "the problem of evil." Briefly stated, it is this: If one believes that (1) God is one, (2) God acts in human history, (3) God is all-knowing (omniscient), (4) God is all-powerful (omnipotent), (5) God is good, and yet (6) there is unjustified evil in the world, then one is involved in a self-contradiction. An all-knowing, all-powerful God who is also good, after all, would never allow unjustified evil to exist and would never need to do so for lack of ability to stop it.

Aside from raising a fundamental issue concerning the nature of God, this severely complicates the problem of recognizing when God produces an act, and when not. If we could claim that God does only good, then we would have a clear criterion by which to know when God is acting. Restricting God's action to the good, however, compromises divine unity and power, for who or what else is then responsible for the evil we experience? On the other hand, if God does produce evil, what are we to make of the claim of divine goodness? And how can we know when God has been involved in an act and when not?

To resolve the problem of evil, one must deny—or at least soften—one of the premises listed above. One classical Jewish approach restricted God's power (assumption #4), claiming that "all is in the hands of Heaven except the fear of Heaven."[15] That is, God *could* control everything but *chose* not to do so in order to grant to human beings the freedom to make some decisions and the ability to carry them out.[16] This makes people, rather than God, the culprits for much of the evil we experience in this world while yet explaining how God remains good.[17]

This "free-will defense" for God becomes questionable, though, when innocent people suffer and die in situations where no human will is involved, as in natural disasters such as disease and earthquakes. Some of the damage done by floods, hurricanes, earthquakes, and many diseases results from bad human planning (building homes in a floodplain or on a known earthquake fault, for example), but these natural forces often do their damage regardless of human action. Indeed, it is impossible to live without incurring some such risks. Moreover, even when some people have been irresponsible, many morally good adults and innocent children suffer in the process. How could a good, powerful God allow this?

Because of such weaknesses in this "free-will defense," rabbis and philosophers within the Jewish tradition, in search of other explanations, have some-

times denied or restricted one of the other assumptions entailed in the problem
of evil. So, for example, the Bible and the rabbis of the Talmud variously adjusted
the last assumption, that there is evil in the world. Along these lines, they sometimes claimed that people deserve the suffering they endure, whether or not they
recognize this, and thus the pain they feel, while certainly unpleasant, is not
evil.[18] They also maintained that people pay for the sins of their parents and,
therefore, the suffering, while possibly unmerited by the children, is in the larger
scheme of things retribution for past wrongs.[19] A major rabbinic adjustment of
the last premise was that God rewards and punishes not only in this world but in
a world to come, and there the accounts of unpunished malefactors and
unrewarded benefactors will be rectified. God's justice and goodness are thus
preserved, despite present appearances.[20] Maimonides (1140–1204), following
Augustine, even went so far as to deny existence to evil, maintaining that it is
only the absence of good.[21] However difficult this idea may be to swallow in the
face of the pain felt by many, it too rescues God from responsibility for evil. If
there is no evil, nobody can be blamed for it!

Jewish naturalists like Mordecai M. Kaplan (1881–1983), Milton Steinberg
(1903–1950), and Harold Kushner (1935–) have instead preferred to restrict
God's actions to the good, consciously giving up God's omnipotence in the process. Thus, Kaplan claims that "earthquakes and volcanic eruptions, devastating storms and floods, famines and plagues, noxious plants and animals . . . are
simply that phase of the universe which has not yet been completely penetrated
by godhood," for "the modern conception of God" follows the less frequent rabbinic opinion, according to which "The Holy One, blessed be He, does not associate His name with evil, but only associates it with that which is good."[22]
Similarly, Harold Kushner, in a moving popular book, has maintained that all
excuses for an omnipotent God become untenable in the face of senseless personal tragedy and that we must consequently affirm that God, though good, is
not all-powerful.[23]

Even Kaplan, though, admits that his position "involves a radical change
in the traditional concept of God" because it undermines divine omnipotence
and omniscience.[24] It also understates the reality of evil. Kaplan specifically affirms that evils exist,[25] but it is hard to take them seriously if the power of God
is behind the good but does not participate in perpetrating evil. God, after all,
is our symbol for ultimate reality. Therefore, restricting God to the good, as
Kaplan and Kushner have done, makes evil metaphysically unreal. We might
wish this were so, and we might warm to thinkers who tell us that it is. But ultimately this only deceives us, for evil is as real, as permanent, and as powerful a
part of our experience as good is. It therefore behooves us to build that reality
into our conception of God.

Of the various ways of doing so, the extreme positions on both ends of the spectrum were already articulated in ancient times. One is that we must simply accept the evil we experience as an act of God that we cannot understand.[26]

The opposite position, that there is no God who enforces the rules of justice, was classified as foolish and heretical in classical Jewish literature but can no longer be cavalierly dismissed. Richard Rubenstein has argued that the Holocaust demonstrates once and for all that there is no God who acts in history, that there is only the overpowering, amoral God of nature. In my view, Rubenstein underestimates the positive experiences of life, and his theory wreaks havoc with our moral expectations and practice—both of which are equally part of the world we know—but he has courageously forced his readers to focus on the hard realities at the core of this prime objection to theism.[27]

Between these extremes, a variety of positions have been proposed. Each shies away from divorcing God from evil, on the one hand, and from making God amoral, on the other. Typical of intermediate stances on any issue, these positions lack the conceptual cleanness of the extreme views described above, but they capture more of the intellectually messy reality of our experience. In that sense, they are probably closer to the truth.

My own position, developed fully in my book on Jewish theology,[28] maintains that to resolve the intellectual problem of evil we must differentiate between two meanings of "God" that the Jewish tradition conflated: God as the powers beyond our understanding or control, and God as the paradigm and support for goodness and justice. When the term "God" denotes the powers that we experience in life beyond our understanding or control, God definitely is involved in undeserved human suffering.

The Jewish tradition did not shrink from this. The rabbis even claimed that Jews must *thank* God for whatever evil befalls them and not just for the good things they enjoy:

> Do not behave towards Me as the heathens behave toward their gods. When happiness comes to them, they sing praises to their gods . . . but when retribution comes upon them they curse their gods. . . . If I bring happiness upon you give thanks, and when I bring sufferings give thanks also.[29]

The rabbis went further yet: Jews must *bless* God for evil as they bless God for good, as an expression of our love of God.[30] To do otherwise would compromise God's unity:

> "I, even I, am He, and there is no God in addition to me; it is I that kill, and it is I that make alive; I wound and I heal" (Deuteronomy 32:39). This verse is an answer to those who say, "There is no Power in heaven," or to those who say "There are two Powers in heaven," or to those who say, "There is no Power who can make alive or kill, do evil or do good."[31]

On the other hand, when the word "God" denotes the paradigm and support for justice and goodness, God certainly is *not* involved in undeserved suffering. Just as much as the rabbis—and I—acknowledge that evil and suffering occur in our lives, honesty requires us to recognize also that much undeserved blessing occurs in our lives. We may be more aware of God when things are not going well for us; we notice our skin, for example, only when it is cut, bruised, or burned. This, however, is a fault in our cognizance, for God is present in our ongoing sustenance and well-being at least as much as in our privations and distress. Indeed, the Jewish tradition, by claiming that God's chief attribute is goodness[32] and that we must bless God a hundred times each day,[33] asserted that, on balance, we have much more to thank God for than to complain about.[34] The Jewish assumption that God is good and just is so deeply rooted that, throughout history, Jews have protested vehemently and eloquently whenever events reveal God to be unjust or malevolent.[35] Such protest makes sense only if one first assumes that God can be expected to be just and good. We must, in any case, note and appreciate God's presence in the good as much as we cry out and protest to God for the bad.

The tradition conflated these meanings of "God" as a statement of faith: In the future, power would be consistently united with goodness. By acknowledging the many cases in which that does not happen in life as we know it, though, and by insisting that the Messiah has yet to come, the tradition affirmed that that exclusive linkage of power to goodness would take place in the future. In the meantime, we must still believe that justice, morality, and compassion are crucial, even if they are not rewarded.[36] We simply have to advance our thinking to a point that some of the rabbis had already reached, namely, that doing the right thing for the sake of reward is really not the proper motivation and often does not work out anyway, and that in the end the only reward for doing God's will is the satisfaction of having done so and the impetus to fulfill it yet again.[37]

Responding to People in Their Suffering

The depth of our emotional distress in the face of suffering is at least partially due to our inability to make sense of our pain—especially, for believers, in the presence of a powerful, benevolent God. After all, we are not bifurcated beings; our emotions and our intellects are interrelated. As long as we recognize that rational deliberation can never substitute for the outpouring of emotion required to cope with emotionally trying circumstances, the quest for a theory (such as my attempt to articulate my own above) that adequately accounts for our various experiences in the world, both good and bad, is not only intellectually necessary but emotionally beneficial. Indeed, often the fact that chaplains and other religious people are struggling with these issues is more important than the particular answers given—although, as the Talmud acknowledged in prohibiting visitors from using the theology of Job's friends, some suggested theodicies can be not only theologically suspect, but downright hurtful.

While intellectual wrestling with the phenomenon of suffering can help those in the throes of disease, their emotional needs must also be met directly. Sufferers can now be assisted by medication to cope with pain, but for a variety of reasons, American physicians often do not provide sufficient medication to quell pain.[38] Judaism's view of pain as something to be avoided would urge that physicians pay more attention to helping their patients in this way.

The Jewish tradition, though, recognized that medical suffering comes from other factors as well. Thus according to Jewish law, when one person assaults another, the assailant must not only pay for the medical expenses, time lost, and the loss in income, but also, as separate sums, for the pain and embarrassment of the injury. The payment for pain is measured in a way that recognizes that people feel pain in varying ways and degrees. The payment for embarrassment is assessed according to how the victim's status was diminished by the injury in his or her own eyes and in the estimation of the community. Moreover, paying the fine is not enough; the assailant must also ask forgiveness from the victim.[39]

While these laws apply to cases of assault, they articulate aspects of medical suffering even when the illness was not intentionally caused by other people. Illness by its very nature is degrading. Things that you could easily do before you can no longer do. Some people even lose control of their bodily functions.

In addition to embarrassment, loneliness is another critical factor in medical suffering. When you cannot interact with people in the ways and in the settings you and they are used to, you are not sure what to talk about. Moreover, friends and family, instead of seeing you in the usual places, must go to the antiseptic atmosphere of a hospital or nursing home, whose sights and smells uncomfortably reinforce their own sense of vulnerability. No wonder they seldom come.

To cope with the embarrassment and loneliness involved in illness, the Jewish tradition has developed several strategies: the commandment to visit the sick, prayer, and ethical wills.

Ill people are not simply physical organisms afflicted with a virus or bacterium; they are whole human beings. Thus even if medicine cannot cure the person, we collectively have the duty to attend to his or her emotional, psychological, and social well-being. As the *Zohar*, a thirteenth-century work of Jewish mysticism, says, "If a physician cannot give his patient medicine for his body, he should [at least] make sure that medicine is given him for his soul."[40] Visiting the sick (*biqqur holim*) is a religious requirement of every Jew (not just the rabbi, doctor, or nurse).[41] Therefore, at least as early as the fourteenth century, and continuing today in many contemporary congregations of all denominations, synagogues have established Biqqur Holim societies, consisting of members who have taken it upon themselves to make sure that sick people are visited, whether they have family doing that or not.[42]

While visiting the sick primarily provides emotional and social support to the ailing, it can affect the person's physical status as well. Certainly those who are visited often have much more motivation to fight to overcome their disease, for it is clear that others want them to survive. As the Talmud says:

> Rabbi Abba son of Rabbi Hanina said: He who visits an invalid takes away a sixtieth of his pain [or, in another version, a sixtieth of his illness] . . .
>
> When Rabbi Dimi came [from Palestine], he said: He who visits the sick causes him to live, while he who does not causes him to die. How does he cause this? . . . He who visits the sick prays that he may live . . . [while] he who does not visit the sick prays neither that he may live nor die.[43]

The Talmud here is asserting two aspects of the spiritual elements of recovery. On a social plane, those who visit the sick help to shift the patient's focus from the pain and degradation of the illness to the joy of the company of friends and family. They thus take away a sixtieth of the pain of the illness. Visitors also reassure the patient that family and friends are keenly interested in their recovery, and they remind the patient of life outside the sickroom. They thereby reinforce the patient's determination to overcome the illness altogether or at least as many of its effects as they can. Visitors are thus instrumental in motivating the patient to follow a medical regimen of healing, however tedious or painful it may be, and so, in the Talmud's alternative reading, they effectively take away a sixtieth of the patient's illness itself.

Visitors affect the patient on a more religious plane as well. By praying for the patient, and by indicating that prayers are being offered in the synagogue on his or her behalf, visitors invoke the aid of God, the ultimate Healer. Jewish prayer is traditionally done in community, in part because Jewish sources maintain that communal prayer convinces God to grant a request more effectively than private prayer does.[44] Visitors' prayers and those recited in the synagogue on behalf of the patient thus throw the weight of the entire community behind the patient's own plea to God for recovery.

As we have noted above, the tradition links sickness with sin, and so the Talmud records this remark by Rabbi Alexandri in the name of Rabbi Hiyya bar Abba: "A sick person does not recover from illness until all his/her sins are forgiven, as [the juxtaposition in the following verse shows, for] it is written, 'God forgives all your sins, God heals all your diseases' (Psalms 103:3)."[45] Jewish confessional prayers, though, are expressed in the first-person plural, for Jewish sources maintain that requests for forgiveness are most effective when *we* recite them as part of a community rather than when *I* recite them by myself.[46] Praying for the sick may thus alleviate feelings of guilt connected with the disease, for now the entire community is asking for both forgiveness and healing.

Visitors must also pay attention to the physical needs of the sick. Thus the Talmud tells the following story:

> Rabbi Helbo fell ill. Rabbi Kahana then went [to the house of study] and proclaimed, "Rabbi Helbo is ill." Nobody, however, visited him. Rabbi Kahana rebuked them [the disciples], saying, "Did it ever happen that one of Rabbi Akiba's students fell ill, and the [rest of the] disciples did not visit him?" So Rabbi Akiba himself entered [Rabbi Helbo's house] to visit him, and because they swept and sprinkled the ground before him [that is, cleaned the house and put it in order], Rabbi Helbo recovered. Rabbi Akiba then went forth and lectured: He who does not visit the sick is like one who sheds blood.[47]

Taking physical care of the sick can include not only cleaning house, but shopping for groceries, doing laundry, taking over carpool duties, and seeing to the other needs of the patient's children. Depending upon the circumstances, it can also include more direct physical interventions like taking the patient for a ride in a wheelchair, feeding the patient, and attending to the patient's other physical needs.

Mostly, though, visiting the sick involves talking with the patient, and that is what often causes the greatest degree of discomfort. Those who visit the sick often do not know what to say or do. Some would rather not hear about the patient's aches and pains, much less about a painful or dangerous procedure the patient just endured or is facing, because such talk makes them sad and engenders thoughts about their own vulnerability. The food served at the facility and the weather quickly lose their interest as topics of conversation. Since few of us are trained in effective visiting techniques, visitors soon feel frustrated in their desires to help and support the patient. All of these feelings deter people from visiting the sick any more than they feel they absolutely must.

The Jewish tradition has some practical advice for making such visits more pleasant and effective.[48] So, for example, Jewish sources are aware of the fact that visitors who stand or sit higher than the patient's head accentuate the patient's incapacity in comparison to their able-bodied state. They also make the patient look up to them, thus further symbolizing a gap in status. To avoid these feelings, visitors should sit at the same level as the patient's head so that their relative heights communicate equality and support.[49]

In addition to praying with the patient, family visitors should raise some practical topics. Specifically, if patients have not previously filled out a will or a living will for health care, they should be asked to specify their wishes about the disposition of their property and the course of their medical treatment.

In addition, visitors can help a patient complete an ethical will, a document developed in the Middle Ages by the Jewish community in which a patient tells some of the family history and expresses his or her feelings for friends and relatives, values, and hopes. In times past, this was usually done in the form of a letter, but now patients often tape their remarks. Visitors can help them by asking leading questions, especially with regard to the patient's memories of the past. Children and, especially, grandchildren will be thrilled to have this document, and creating it provides an important task for patients who cannot do much else. Moreover, since perfectly healthy people create living wills, it reunites the sick with the well, giving them a sense of worth and belonging.

Most time spent with the patient, though, does not lend itself to discussion of specific decisions or projects. How, then, should visitors fill the time of their visit?

Jewish legal sources are silent about this, but Jewish theological concepts provide important clues. Every human being, according to the Torah, bears the dignity of being created in the image of God. Since illness is inherently degrading, the key to speaking with sick people is to bolster that sense of worth. Visitors must be especially on guard to avoid infantilizing the patient, for talking down to the patient reinforces his or her sense of loss of power and honor. Visitors should rather engage the patient in conversations on the level and subjects of the patient's normal interests. Indeed, one of the most enlightening experiences of my early rabbinic career was giving a series of lectures on Jewish theology to residents of a Jewish nursing home. They were all college graduates who had never studied theology before, but who relished intellectual discussions and who, frankly, were bored with bingo. Visitors do not normally discuss Jewish theology but, as I learned to my surprise, conversations with patients can and should be challenging, covering a wide variety of topics. The very normalcy of such discussions communicates that the illness has not diminished the visitor's respect for the patient's intelligence and humanity.

Implications for Medicine, Medical Education, and Bioethics

Facing medical suffering in a theological context, as I have done above, has important implications for the practice of medicine and for the education of future doctors and nurses. In the context of American medicine, where the body is generally seen as a machine that needs to be fixed, by far the most important implication of this study is that medical personnel must learn to see people as people. The legal need to pay attention to patients' medical choices has alerted physicians to the varying moral stances that people have; the phenomena of medical suffering should inform them of their histories, communities, hopes, and fears as well. Except for pain control, medical personnel need not have an expertise in these matters, but they must recognize them for the serious factors that they are and learn how to consult others who do know how to help patients with them—clergy, social workers, and the family themselves. Since these factors critically affect the patient's willingness to cooperate with a medical regimen and, indeed, his or her will to live, failing to acknowledge these factors and to find means to deal with them can undermine any medical treatment. Medical personnel are therefore not just being nice in seeking to alleviate the nonmedical aspects of medical suffering; they are simply being good doctors and nurses.

Similarly, bioethics can no longer limit itself to the physical factors of medical care. As a field, bioethics in recent years has expanded its horizons from issues arising out of the medical care of specific patients to the broader context of prevention of disease and the distribution of medical care. This study, and indeed this book, is one effort in the drive to expand bioethics yet further, recognizing the "soft" factors that crucially affect the health of individual patients and of society as a whole. Patients' beliefs, fears, and hopes enter the hospital with them and affect their behavior before and after their hospital stay. Whether a person seeks to alleviate suffering with drugs or alcohol or in more healthful ways is often a product of such "soft" factors, and the course of a person's disease often depends on them as well. Adequate bioethics then, like adequate medicine, depends on taking these factors into account.

This, of course, is not good news to either medical personnel or bioethicists, for it makes their jobs even harder. Actually, these factors have been playing a role in their fields all along; it is just that now we are confronting them more fully. Instead of pretending that patients preserve their health or recover from illness on the basis of physical factors alone, it will ultimately help everybody to acknowledge the utter ambiguity and insecurity of our existence, not only with a commitment to truth and morality, but with distinctly religious values: faith, strength, wisdom, the willingness to cry when appropriate, a sense of humor, and hope.

9

To Change and to Accept in a Technological Society

Per Anderson

The following prayer, attributed to Reinhold Niebuhr and widely invoked by people facing ordeal, epitomizes the problem that suffering poses for a technological society.

> God, give us grace to accept with serenity the things that cannot be changed, courage to change the things which should be changed, and the wisdom to distinguish the one from the other.[1]

Suffering descends, variously yet eventually, on all of us. What suffering means to us, however, and what we do in response are profoundly informed by a now well-established way of life that denies us the critical powers that the Niebuhr prayer seeks. As a stance toward suffering, the prayer is in some way intuitively plausible, as its enduring popularity confirms. But its currency also points to a persistent need for such an entreaty.

Suffering requires different responses to its various sources, but the morality sought by the prayer—particularly, the serenity to accept and the wisdom to distinguish—is alien to the habits of thought and action typical of technological life. Acceptance and change as general orientations seem to many to be mutually exclusive. Yet the prayer has plausibility, in part, because the norms of technological life are no longer unimpeachable bases for thinking about and responding to suffering. Long-standing worries about the moral ambiguity of technological society enjoy increasing recognition today,[2] even as the beat of technological progress goes on. If technology promises to save us from suffering, experience seems to teach us that it does not succeed.

In this chapter, I support a stance toward suffering that is something like the prayer. I do so by examining the different problems of and responses to suffering operative in the prayer and by arguing that cultural authority for change at the exclusion of the acceptance of suffering cannot be justified. In defense of the Niebuhr prayer and building upon certain assumptions about the social role of technology,[3] I seek to show how technology launches its own distinctive problem of suffering, one no less vexing and persistent than the theological version that most Westerners know: "Why, God?" A credible solution to the technological problem of suffering is nowhere to be seen, but simply noting and examining the problem are appropriate first steps.

If, as Emmanuel Levinas contends, the "why?" response to suffering has been constitutive of Western consciousness until this century, we would do well to think about our technological problem of suffering against the background of "classic theodicy, which reflects this consciousness."[4] Analysis of the classic problem can also support reflection on the acceptance of suffering, a notion that the technological problem may require us to retrieve. Despite being eclipsed by technology, traditional Western theodicy may bear some wisdom for a new ethic of acceptance.[5] Classic theodicy has been a condition for the possibility of accepting what cannot be changed, and this response may have a legitimate place in technological life.

To think about and name the problem of suffering, I shall employ the heuristic potential of ideal types. Theodicies are always particular in form, use, and result. Yet, the examination of any particular depends on some fictive construct that illuminates the particular through comparative reference. Thought and discourse depend on ideal type categories. Further, the use of ideal type "responses" to suffering will enable us to see how medicine (as technology) meets religion on the question of suffering. This is a virtue of the Niebuhr prayer. Reflective of our technological situation, the prayer frames suffering in practical terms; thus, both technological and classic religious responses to suffering can be compared and better understood. What surgeons and pastors typically do in response to suffering can be illuminated and related by posing the question of normative response.[6] How should we respond to suffering?

Chaos, Refusal, and Anguish: The Nature of Suffering

The question of a fitting response to suffering assumes some understanding of its nature. Although suffering varies, there appear to be common structural elements of cause, manifestation, and amelioration that justify one category for the many. Recent interpreters tend to agree that serious suffering is a place apart from the ordered, paramount realities or worlds that constitute human identity.[7] Sufferers want a way out of these alien places or a way to remake them.

Suffering is a distinctly human experience wherein a person is acted upon in a way that threatens or destroys the integrity of the self. That which constitutes the self is always vulnerable to unwelcome change. The human ability to envisage a future sponsors constant anxiety about the loss of integrity, which can reach a threshold of intensity at which suffering occurs. This threshold varies from person to person, as do the parts of the self that fall prey to change. But, in one way or another, suffering occurs when unwelcome and intolerable change, relative to the particularities of self and society, throws the self into a chaotic state of loss, alienation, and terror about an uncertain future. The question so often voiced by the sufferer, "What did I do to deserve this?" testifies to the shock of difference born of the negation of a preferred way of being. Some crucial aspect of self and world—a relation, a possession, a project—fails under some opposing power. To this, the self can only say No! in self-affirmation and protest. Such refusal of suffering bespeaks a break, not simply a low point, in a life story. Serious suffering is a form of death.[8]

Suffering, then, is no place to live. Purpose and orientation fall before betrayal or ignorance or disease. Suffering's ability to frustrate autonomous action convinced H. Richard Niebuhr that persons live more by their responses to action upon them than by their pursuit of ends or conformity to law. Humans live always in a mode of response to action upon the self and anticipation of that response.[9] As Eric Cassell and others describe it, suffering befalls the self from beyond and renders it passive.[10] This imposition results in what Cassell terms "self-conflict." The shattered-world character of suffering means scandal, the uncanny, the unassumable. Once past the shock of chaos and the defiance of refusal, the self recoils in anguish:

> I am at an impasse, and you, O God, have brought me here. From my earliest days, I heard of you. From my earliest days, I believed in you. . . . For me, your yoke was easy. On me your presence smiled.
> Noon has darkened. As fast as she could say, "He's dead," the light dimmed. And where are you in this darkness? I learned to spy you in the light. Here in this darkness I cannot find you. If I had never looked for you, or looked but never found, I would not feel this pain of your absence. Or is it not your absence in which I dwell but your elusive troubling presence?
> Will my eyes adjust to this darkness? Will I find you in the dark—not in the streaks of light which remain, but in the darkness?[11]

Just as suffering is always individual, so too are the manifestations of self-conflict. Any constitutive relation of self—body, spirit, nature, the neighbor, the ultimate—can be the site of suffering. Struggle over loss of bodily limb and a passion for its use can provoke suffering, as can a child's death in a world governed by divine power and love. Because it is particular and unique, suffering resists understanding and fitting response. Those who suffer typically feel alone, beyond the reach even of sympathetic others.[12]

Although people suffer differently, we cannot overlook the ongoing participation and formation of persons in cultural systems that provide relatively common worlds of belief, value, and practice that condition any experience of suffering. Because humans have a social nature, we share social meanings of suffering. Given the power of suffering to crush life, and given the interests of groups in affirming and perpetuating themselves, we might expect that all social groups continually engage the problem of suffering. For Peter Berger, societies are always involved in processes of "nomization," intended to provide meaningful order to human experience (something animals need not do). This socially constructed nomos is always vulnerable to suffering, which has the power to discredit social orders as well as to defeat individuals. As part of its social nature, the self takes from its primary society some world and some strategy for the maintenance of that world in the face of chaos.[13] This is the basic function of "theodicy," conventionally defined: to reconcile the ways of God to humanity and to restore to consistency—and thus order—a set of claims about God and world. Theodicy involves some explanation or interpretation of suffering and some justification or evaluation of that explanation.

With Berger's social theory, we can think of theodicy in terms more expansive than conventional parlance. All social ordering, for Berger, represents an implicit form of theodicy in the sense that it seeks to clothe the individual in an all-embracing fabric of meanings and thus to encompass both the good and the bad. By adopting these meanings, the individual transcends her or his own uniqueness, including the uniqueness of suffering. The individual faces these realities in the company of the group by participating in a larger nomos.

> He sees himself "correctly," that is, within the co-ordinates of reality as defined by his society. He is made capable of suffering "correctly" and, if all goes well, he may eventually have a "correct" death (or a "good death," as it used to be called). In other words, he may "lose himself" in the meaning-giving nomos of his society. In consequence, the pain becomes more tolerable, the terror less overwhelming, as the sheltering canopy of the nomos extends to cover even those experiences that may reduce the individual to howling animality.[14]

This formulation accommodates diverse ways of constructing the "problem" of suffering as such and of addressing that problem. Following Berger and given the significance of suffering in individual experience, we should expect a cultural system to provide its participants with some meanings for their encounters with suffering and some strategy for remaking their worlds when they break. Individuals deal with suffering differently, but they do so informed by shared conventional wisdom. Cultural systems, then, typically confer upon individuals some sense of the problem of suffering and some sense of how to respond when suffering comes.

These systems also change. The social role that explicit theological explanations of suffering once played in Western experience—"theodicy" came into the language with Gottfried Leibniz in 1710—may now be eclipsed by other social meanings. What the Christian worldview was for Leibniz's theodicy may now be succeeded by some other "faith" with some other theodicy.

Suffering is experience with a basic structure that takes countless actual forms; these forms are also the stuff of cultural systems. Humans never suffer radically alone. Moments of self-conflict and refusal are conditioned by the socially grounded interpretive apparatus we bring to experience. In this way, the "problem" of suffering, like the particular response it elicits, should be understood as a cultural form.

Further, there is much travail that humans negotiate *without* suffering because the social order gives it a common meaning. For example, the death of a young person in the "prime" of life is usually a different matter for all involved than death at the end of a "full" life; theodicy is at work in the basic social processes that condition the sermon preached at the funeral. Or consider the cancer patient who ceases to ask "What did I do to deserve this?" because her oncologist can promise a near-certain cure. Theodicy, as Berger shows, is a more complex and ordinary process than the explicit religious explanations that we associate with Leibniz's word.

Accepting Suffering:
Classic Theodicy in Form and Function

The most important historical consequence of the disintegration of Christian theodicy in the consciousness of Western [people] has . . . been the inauguration of an age of revolution. History and human action in history have become the dominant instrumentalities by which the nomization of suffering and evil is to be sought. Not submission to the will of God, not hope mediated through the figure of Christ, not expectation of a divinely effected *eschaton* serve any longer to assuage most [people's] anguish.[15]

In American life today, religious belief and practice are no longer the primary means for the nomization of suffering. Technology in general—and medicine especially—fills this social role, and with it comes a decisive shift in human response to suffering. In this section, we shall examine a response with no proper place in the technological society, namely, acceptance. Whether there are good reasons for the crisis of plausibility that besets acceptance is not yet at issue. First, we need to consider what acceptance has meant in Western Christian experience and how it was grounded and formed. For this, we shall consider an ideal type account of "classic theodicy." In a context of some doubt about technological life, sympathetic interpretation may yield insight worthy of retrieval.

If, as Berger contends, modern Western people order suffering through practical action, we might expect attendant doubts about classic theodicy to be moral in nature. In large part, they are. However, the questions and answers of classic theodicy are noetic, manifestations of an anthropology that cannot tolerate chronic chaos insofar as it defeats human interest and ability to construe a world. In suffering, the human meets the uncanny and finds discredited and inoperable the assets by which the world makes sense. As H. Richard Niebuhr contends:

> Whatever else we may need to say about ourselves in defining ourselves, we shall need . . . always to say that we are characterized by awareness and that this awareness is more or less that of intelligence which identifies, compares, analyzes, and relates events so that they come to us not as brute actions, but as understood and as having meaning. . . . But more complexly, we interpret the things that force themselves upon us as parts of wholes, as related and as symbolic of larger meanings. And these larger patterns of interpretation we employ seem to determine—though in no mechanical way—our responses to action upon us.[16]

Niebuhr here captures the basic burden of classic theodicy, namely, to authorize an acceptance of the world—suffering and all—as a divinely ordered cosmos wherein everything has a place and a meaning. Underlying classic theodicy is a worldview that must see suffering in relation to the whole. Put more strongly, suffering must be integral to the whole, part of a good world where there is no pointless suffering and where good finally will triumph over evil. Such is the basic faith of classic theodicy, from Job's comforters to Augustine to John Paul II. Because such global interpretation makes a difference in human response, the presumed intelligibility and purpose of suffering create the possibility of Reinhold Niebuhr's serenity to accept.

The classic response arises from the human need for a nomos wedded to a particular monotheistic worldview. If believed, this outlook always conditions the experience of suffering. In most formulations of the problem, the scandal of suffering stems from the apparent incompatibility of the negative (disease, bondage, abandonment, death) with divine goodness and power. At least since Epicurus, such worldly evil has been a problem for belief in an omnibenevolent, omnipotent, and omniscient God. Since nothing can oppose this God's will, the fact of the negative seems impossible, and yet it exists. The "why?" question both acknowledges the reality of suffering in human life and seeks a source. As Paul Ricoeur observes, classic theodicy seeks an "origin to be discovered."[17]

This standard account needs to be modified in two ways. First, classic ideas about God—especially the idea of the omnipotence of God—condition the classic problem and its resolution. Only a God of power can secure the triumph of the good. The scandal of suffering in Christianity is finally cosmological, arising out of an affirmation of the goodness of creation. Expectations of earthly well-being legitimate the shock of suffering. Whatever the doctrine of God, Christianity affirms both the proper goodness of creation and the reality of temporal agony. This antithesis is the source of the classic self-conflict of Christian suffering.[18]

Second, the problem of theodicy, especially since the Enlightenment, is often understood to be an abstract philosophical problem that threatens the reasonableness of belief in God. Though radical suffering may be a major source of modern atheism, the classical problem speaks to an existential crisis, a broken world in which one cannot live. From this place of self-conflict and refusal, Augustine gives voice to the classic question born of a traditional Christian worldview: "Whence then is evil, since God who is good made all things good? It was the greater and supreme Good who made these lesser goods, but Creator and Creation are alike good. Whence then comes evil?"[19]

From this question of origin, classic theodicy offers a hermeneutical response to suffering, with two aims. First, it seeks to explain (literally) the historical and metaphysical conditions for the possibility of the negative in the world and how the world is as it is. Theodicy here gives suffering "meaning" by providing an all-embracing account of the whole and of the place of the negative in it. Second, beyond the effort to render suffering intelligible as a general phenomenon of the world, classic theodicy seeks to reconcile this apparent evil with a good creation. Thus, it tries to justify (not deny) the evil of suffering through a moral apology for the "value" of the whole. If the negative shatters worlds and leaves people in the chaos of suffering, the traditional hermeneutical response attempts to remake the world through reinterpretation and revaluation of the negative in relation to the whole.

Classic theodicy does not try to explain instances of suffering in their uniqueness. The meaning of the particular arises from participation in the general. Yet, because there can be no pointless suffering, a plausible theodicy must account for multiple forms and degrees, which may result in an eclectic theory of divine purpose. Free-will, educative, eschatological, mystery, and communion interpretations may all be employed in a given theodicy.[20] By the same token, one case of meaningless suffering can discredit the whole theory. If classic theodicy cannot order every negative, it cannot integrate any. For this reason, the suffering of the innocent—especially children—is a perennial challenge to classic theodicy going back to Augustine.

Traditional theodicy rejects the notion that the "goodness" of God and the world can be reconciled with suffering only through equivocation. Further, it denies that a good God and a good world must exclude all negatives. The question is whether the experience that provokes suffering can be purposive in the sense of participating in a good whole. Classic theodicy argues for a transvaluation of suffering in view of its divinely created relation to a greater good. The sources of suffering are said to bear instrumental value, which may be invisible in the situation but visible from a larger frame of reference that changes the moral quality of the particular suffering in question. Classic theodicy puts the burden of justifying instances of suffering upon the moral quality of the whole. Once the source of suffering has been placed within a plausible account of world process, the second and crucial dimension of theodicy involves a moral apology for that process. If this cosmological argument persuades the refusing subject of suffering, a moral order will be apparent. God and the world will appear good for the human being despite evil—and a remaking of the world can follow. Consider two contemporary voices, John Hick and Pope John Paul II:

> Christian theodicy claims . . . that the end to which God is leading us is a good so great as to justify the failures and suffering and sorrow that will have been endured along the way to it. The life of the Kingdom of God will be an infinite, because eternal, good, outweighing all temporal and therefore finite evils. We cannot visualize the life of the redeemed and perfected creation, for all our imagery is necessarily drawn from the present "fallen" world. We can think only in very general terms of the opening up before us of new dimensions of reality.[21]

> Suffering is in itself an experience of evil. But Christ has made suffering the firmest basis of the definitive good, namely the good of eternal salvation. By his suffering on the cross, Christ reached the very roots of evil, of sin and death. He conquered the author of evil, Satan, and his permanent rebellion against the Creator. To the suffering brother or sister Christ discloses and gradually reveals the horizons of the kingdom of God: the horizons of a world converted to the Creator, of a world free from sin, a world being built on the saving power of love. And slowly but effectively, Christ leads into this world, into this kingdom of the Father, suffering man, in a certain sense through the very heart of his suffering.[22]

Classic theodicy undertakes an explanatory and evaluative apology, which aims to resolve the chaos of suffering at the level of the whole by enabling the refusing, conflicted self to integrate the concrete and the particular into a larger worldview of meaning and value. If a given theodicy succeeds, it allows the anomic self to reinterpret and reevaluate the "No." Since classic theodicy is a hermeneutical response, it does not reduce or remove suffering by ending pain or restoring loss. Rather, it responds to the self's loss of self-direction with the power of rational understanding. Still, there is a practical aim: to show the self a way back to a life where the negative can be understood and borne.[23]

Is this understanding and bearing of suffering the serenity with which one accepts "the things that cannot be changed"? And how does classic theodicy deal with "the things that should be changed"? Because the classic response focuses the problem of suffering on the whole, it encourages a faith in reality that justifies a global "Yes" to the fact of suffering. This acceptance—if internalized by the self—must surely alter or transfigure every particular encounter with suffering, even those that clearly should not be accepted, like the lacerations of moral evil. For classic theodicy, some of life's suffering is clearly evil and should be refused, here and now. Still, even in the case of sin or the suffering of the innocent, there is a place in classic theodicy for its ultimate acceptance. In the end, such evil is not really evil because it can be or will be justified in relation to a transcendent good. This good is the work of God, who must be omnipotent in order to secure its actualization.

Global acceptance of suffering is a clear implication of classic theodicy. This serenity to accept is a dispositional ethic that anticipates the reality of the negative: It happens. Suffering, whenever it occurs, involves something that rules the self and "cannot be changed." But the self, while it cannot do anything about this imposition, need not be destroyed. Purposeful suffering can be managed. People can alter attitudes and expectations and so alter the experience of action upon them. Classic theodicy offers the possibility of bearing negatives and, thus, transcending suffering.

But do attitudes and expectations that make suffering bearable also work to undermine a disposition "to change the things that should be changed"? The answer depends on the particular interpretation of suffering that a given theodicy provides. Any classic theodicy ought to provide an interpretive scheme that allows both the subject and the onlooker of suffering to distinguish among experiences of suffering and their sources and to respond appropriately. But the notion of changing what should be changed is clearly not at home in traditional theodicy's moral world, where the issue is more simply to act in conformity with God's will through grace. If God wills that the needs of a neighbor be met, then beneficent acts, which may result in relief of suffering, are required. But such acts may not yield effective change, for change depends on forces that include but largely transcend the human. The human task is fidelity, to do God's will as one can, come what may.

To ask classic theodicy whether its stance toward suffering undermines change begs the question of human responsibility. The impulse to explain suffering assumes that its sources are a given of human life. Traditional theodicy proffers an altered experience of suffering, but not its elimination. Dorothee Soelle captures a crucial conviction of theodicy when she concludes, "Almost all Christian interpretations . . . ignore the distinction between suffering that we can and cannot end."[24] This is another way of noting that for classic theodicy the problem of suffering is finally God's, both as source and solution. Humans should be obedient to God, and God is the beginning and end of suffering. Thus does classic theodicy frame the question of human alteration of a suffering world. Classic theodicy does not glory in suffering. It believes that humans cannot do much to eliminate suffering, but that a suffering world can be rendered bearable.

In sum, classic theodicy is a hermeneutical response to suffering that offers meaning and value in suffering. Suffering can be comprehended and endured because it participates in a wider cosmos made good by an omnipotent and redemptive God. The human task is to discern this order and to live receptively.

Humans can do little about the reality and redemption of suffering, save to view them in a way that lowers the terror. This does not mean fatalism in the face of suffering. While human action cannot save, human action can diminish—or increase—the temporal course of suffering.

Changing the World:
Practical Theodicy in the Technological Society

Let me suggest that the bad things that happen to us in our lives do not have a meaning when they happen to us. They do not happen for any good reason that would cause us to accept them willingly. But we can give them a meaning. We can redeem these tragedies from senselessness by imposing meaning on them.[25]

A prerequisite for such work is the conviction that we live in a world that can be changed. Anyone who lives in a static world view, in a post-figurative culture, that is, one that is intent upon imitation and repetition of the past . . . cannot see learning and change as the most important things one can achieve in life. His attitude toward suffering cannot get beyond acceptance and resignation. Only where change itself is comprehended as an essential human value and acknowledged by society, only there can the passive attitude toward suffering change.[26]

For a technological society, as for classic theodicy, suffering is both vitalizing scandal and abiding reality. Chaos invades a world, and an occasion for remaking arises yet again. But the nomoi that suffering assaults in a technological society are different from those of classic theodicy, as are the attendant responses. Suffering for such a society does not call forth an account of metaphysical origins. It does not subvert faith in a loving God. Rather, suffering evokes rededication to altering a world that can be changed.

It is difficult to specify precisely the advent of advanced technology. In the American context, technology now constitutes what Arthur Melzer terms the "whole purposive structure" of society that produces the "horizon in which every other thing finds its place."[27] It functions as collective ethic and guarantor of the modern world, provides an overarching symbolic frame of reference or world picture for engaging reality, and forms the principal human world. It is our universal cultural system.[28] Technology, therefore, always contends with suffering and so functions as the new theodicy of modern Western societies, a successor to premodern classic theodicy. That is, the powers of technology bear principal responsibility for maintaining the sheltering nomos against chaos.

Modern technology is a practical, collective way of being which glories in creativity and change for the sake of constant progress in a perennial enterprise

of enhancing and extending human capacities and powers. In opposition to presumed limits to the human condition, technology seeks to expand the realm of
human possibility—in the body, in society, in nature.[29] While all humans do this,
modern technology is a unique form of the expansive impulse with unprecedented
traits and implications.[30] Beyond the perennial activity of creating artifacts (tools
and methods), the modern way of being attempts to order all aspects of the world
according to values of efficiency, ease, comfort, and security. Through practical
knowledge and aggressive intervention, technology seeks a world available at
our beck and call.[31] It is

> a way of thinking and believing and feeling, a way of standing in and toward the
> world. Technology . . . is the disposition rationally to order and predict and control
> everything feasible, in order to master fortune and spontaneity, violence and wild-
> ness, and to leave nothing to chance, all in the service of human benefit.[32]

As an enterprise of restless, systematic expansion of autonomous human powers, technology moves against the imposition of alien and unwelcome power—
the human powerlessness—that marks suffering. Technology anticipates and responds to suffering by acting on the concrete and particular things and orders
that threaten or harm the self and its normative world. Technology does not
explain suffering in the world with a view to intrinsic meaning and value; suffering has none. Emmanuel Levinas speaks for this feature of modernity when he
contends that suffering as such is senseless and useless and that its signs of misery
call the Other to help. The self-evident evil of suffering generates practices like
medicine and the "elevated thought of a civilization called to nourish persons
and to lighten their sufferings."[33] Over the course of two centuries, this civilization has come to possess astonishing powers to reduce or remove suffering.

If advanced technology functions as the primary nomos, suffering is more than
personal evil; it is a threat to common order as well. Insofar as technology aims to
reduce or remove suffering, the continued appearance of suffering is a scandal. It
pitches the universe toward chaos and mocks the sufficiency of human instrumentalities. In contemporary life, people afflicted by chronic pain, for example,
carry such chaos. Perhaps because medicine typically does not know what to do
for these patients, they often report misunderstanding and neglect.[34] Chronic
pain is a strange and forbidding world indeed, outside the shelter of the technological universe.

Nevertheless, pain beyond practical remedy must still be refused because it
can still be addressed in some fashion. This, at least, is the modernist self-understanding. To define suffering as senseless and useless, except when undertaken
voluntarily to further its abolition, is to reject the agenda of classic theodicy out
of hand. Some critics question the explanatory adequacy of traditional theodicies
and conclude that these arguments cannot encompass the radical evils of the

twentieth century or the agony of innocents. For, as noted above, if a classic account cannot explain all suffering, it cannot justify any.

Yet, behind this sort of criticism, there often lurks a more basic and devastating critique—like that voiced by Dostoyevsky's Ivan Karamazov or Camus's Dr. Rieux—that rejects any effort to justify any human suffering for a higher good.[35] These voices of "protest" reveal several sources. The anathema on suffering arises clearly from modern worldliness and humanism, but even more decisively from militant convictions about change. Even if suffering cannot be removed by human remedy, it can be reduced—and there is always solidarity. The impulse to justify suffering as a fixture of the universe is merely a remnant of the days of human impotence. The modern protest against theological explanations of suffering arises primarily from moral notions stemming from a basic modern conviction that humans can exercise a practical mode of ordering. As a result of this shift, the response of classic theodicy appears, in principle, to be party to sanctioning the status quo. If practice does not contribute to concrete, historical change, it is morally suspect. Simply by explaining, the classic type of theodicy mediates a moral practice that looks beyond present evil to heaven above. If traditional theodicy licenses a global "Yes" to a suffering world, the technological project assumes a foundational "No." The absurdity of twentieth-century events like the Holocaust reinforces this anathema against explanation.[36]

The evil of justification assumes a militantly melioristic sense of life, nourished by the awesome gains of modern technology. As we readily see in the ever expanding powers of medicine, technology proceeds as if all suffering can be overcome; every achievement confirms and heightens expectations. The search for meaning in suffering seems a misplaced rationality that admits something technology addresses with systematic denial. To strive to remove or reduce suffering and then seek meaning for that which practice cannot change misses the point of technology. The protest of recent Western philosophy and theology against classic theodicy is basically methodological: The traditional response simply misconstrues suffering. In a world still subject to great evil, if a philosophy or theology of suffering does not "allow the screams of our society to be heard," it fails a basic moral test and must be vigorously rejected.[37]

With technology as theodicy, a practical ethic of suffering, wedded to a theology of worldly redemption, has become an authoritative option in contemporary Christian reflection on suffering.[38] A God of technology, who opposes suffering and who empowers humans to change it, is the successor to a morally discredited classical theism. Like the structures of technological life, these newer theologies will have nothing to do with explanations that justify suffering. The way that outrage about suffering today unites diverse ideologies marks the cultural significance of technology. This outrage lends energy and focus to practical institutional structures.

The Problem of Technological Suffering: Structural Evil

But what about the persistence of suffering? Are there not limits to the way of technology? We have thus far examined the question of response to suffering in ideal typical terms. These types—classic hermeneutical and technological practical—provide frameworks for thinking about the question. No human lives either "pure" form. I turn now to how we ought to respond to suffering, given diverse options and certain doubts about the adequacy of either type. Aware as we may be of various ways of being, a person must finally live in some particular world at a given time. Even though that world may not structure the whole of one's relations, being related at all means living in one world and not another. Consequently, when we encounter suffering, we construe it and respond from within a particular world.

Clearly, technology is the first world in American society. As Paul Ricoeur notes, suffering is primarily about "a *task* to be accomplished."[39] Remedial action is the preferred mode of response; no one wants it otherwise. As we have noted, modernist thinking about technology insists upon an uncompromising stance—a methodical posture of refusal—which has produced immense powers to act. Looking at the world "as if" suffering need not be has progress on its side. In and through technology, we not only expand the realm of practical possibility, but also experience a concrete validation of scientific-technological beliefs about reality. The cultural place and prestige of technology are not without cause.

Still, recent experiences of technology are not without an ambiguity that may warrant something like Niebuhr's prayer. Before we explore such an alternative to total refusal, we need to note a further reason why the technological posture may be undaunted by the continuing tale of human misery. Consider Camus's Dr. Rieux, who believes himself to be right in fighting the world as he finds it:

"After all," the doctor repeated, then hesitated again, fixing his eyes on Tarrou, "it's something that a man of your sort can understand most likely, but, since the order of the world is shaped by death, mightn't it be better for God if we refuse to believe in Him and struggle with all our might against death, without raising our eyes toward heaven where He sits in silence."

Tarrou nodded.

"Yes. But your victories will never be lasting; that's all."

Rieux's face darkened.

"Yes, I know that. But it's no reason for giving up the struggle."

"No reason, I agree. Only, I now can picture what this plague must mean to you."

"Yes. A never ending defeat."

Tarrou stared at the doctor for a moment, then turned and tramped heavily

toward the door. Rieux followed him and was almost at his side when Tarrou, who
was staring at the floor, suddenly said:
   "Who taught you all of this, doctor?"
   The reply came promptly:
   "Suffering."[40]

Arthur Melzer identifies an element of the technological worldview that explains why classic and technological stances toward suffering are different and
why the modernist can live with the refusal of suffering, without the intelligible
universe of traditional thought. For Melzer, the modern project is not about at-
tainment of the good but about avoidance of evil. Skeptical about the realization
of happiness, modernity has adopted a "negative orientation" toward existence.
Life, as for Hobbes, is endless striving and desiring without repose or possession.
The reality that organizes this striving is death and its derivative evils. Progress
means not approximation of the good but distance from evil.[41] For Rieux, the
ceaseless reality of suffering can be admitted but need not deter a struggle in
which there is nobility and a kind of victory in delaying defeat. Real progress
against suffering can be achieved, even as the hydra-headed monster lives on.
   Without doubt, the modern refusal of death produces powers that we cannot
dismiss without ontological self-contradiction. How many of us owe our lives to
advanced technology? Yet, in our quest for comprehensive mastery, we may be
practicing a stance toward the world that produces evils that sour the goods.
Paradoxically, a project designed to avoid evil may need to reckon with its complicity in the production of evil. If so, what becomes of the legitimacy of this
dominant mode of response to suffering? If these evils are necessary and perhaps
permanent consequences of technology, what are we to do?
   As Leon Kass observes, modern Western societies (unlike the ancients) have
a pact with technology (and not with religion or politics or law) because of a
foundational belief that barriers to happiness arise not from turbulences of the
ego that require healing or governance but from a world stingy with provisions
and threatening to being. Kass wonders whether modern ambitions for environmental mastery are really feasible.[42] Consider Dr. Rieux's sense of "never ending
defeat." Since Jacques Ellul's initial complaints thirty years ago, problems of unintended consequences and of autonomy have both qualified and shaped the
course of technology development.[43] "Progress" in human control of the world
seems to bring with it some new dependence or menace calling for a remedial
response. Such has been the modern experience of technology, which Edward
Tenner sets forth in an account of the "revenge effects" of technology. Embody-
ing a modern sense of nature as our adversary, Tenner's study focuses on "the
tendency of the world around us to get even, to twist our cleverness against us."
Revenge effects operate independently of human intention and refer instead to

"the way reality seems to strike back at our efforts" to control the world. Such defeat has been an abiding fact of modern life.[44]

These dynamics do not deny technology's successes. But do they falsify its dreams of modern mastery of the world? Problems with autonomy and unintended consequences may, in principle, be overcome by improved practice based on greater focus and precision about human well-being. To the degree that these problems stem from minimalist conceptions of the good characteristic of the liberal society, they will not be easily resolved but are not beyond some reform.[45] Remedial practices of assessment and regulation and appeals for responsibility (more and better technique) are typical candidates for the reform of technology. They call for a more sophisticated technology, a wiser assault on the enemy, and "endless rituals of vigilance."[46]

But Tenner's recommendations for a technology less subject to revenge does not anticipate some final victory over nature. Voicing the "negative orientation" of modernity, Tenner regards revenge as a permanent feature of technological gain, meaning that we "must always look back just because reality is indeed gaining on us."[47] Here is technology doing what Melzer thinks it promises: to battle the negative, not to secure happiness. Though liberal moderns agree little about the good, we do agree about opposing the evils of poverty, disease, and death. To the degree that technology fulfills that mission, the "revenge effects" of technology can be viewed as the tragic consequences of a noble battle against a world hostile to humans. We may lament never reaching the promised land of mastery, but we do not stop striving because the goal is unattainable.

But what is to be done about human complicity in this backlash that results from our attempts to change the world? Do we believe the gains of technology on the whole outweigh, and thus justify, the losses? Given decades of critical observation and reflection on technology, it seems reasonable to form some determinant judgments about this way of life. We know it well, and we seem now to know also that the moral ambiguity of technology is not a passing, precritical phase; thus, we cannot look on human complicity with innocent eyes. We do both good and evil with technology, and we know it. We may try to relativize human culpability by reference to a great good, as classic theodicy does, but the production of evil by a project energized by protest against suffering is a situation that must be recognized and engaged. What does technology do about its complicity in suffering?

In addition to unintended consequences, which indicate limits to human mastery of the world, there is another form of moral ambiguity in technology: its effects on the human subject. We know, in countless ways, the gains of technology, how it infuses life with new and seemingly beneficial powers in virtually every sphere. We know that we are so formed by technological dispositions, patterns, and artifacts that we can barely imagine life without them. They constitute personal and cultural identity and are the form and substance of our basic dependencies. Our deep and significant relation to technology is why it condi-tions—perhaps determines—typical modern attitudes, expectations, and prac-tices regarding suffering.

Modern technology provides a vast array of powers to change environmen-tal sources of suffering. We manipulate and create in ways that reduce or remove objective causes. But suffering is more than pain or loss as such. It is an internal disruption of identity and integrity, of self and world, precipitated by external powers that impose themselves, obstructing the purposive unity of the self and resulting in inner conflict. Suffering exists in relation to some reality antithetical to normative self and world. Whether we suffer when faced with chance, limita-tion, toil, disease, or death turns upon our preexisting system of meaning and upon what we then make of the negative.

If "revenge effects" and other types of unintended consequences cannot be overcome by human striving, the modern attempt to master the world for human benefit is a narrative in need of critical examination and revision. Because of the story that we tell in the technological society about self and world and because of the remarkable success of that story, there is an intensity to our suffering that is of our own making. Suffering in the technological society is a keenly miserable experience.

Technology will not make anything of suffering except a better future; suffer-ing is otherwise "useless." But human interaction with and reliance on technol-ogy generates its own kind of suffering when technology cannot remove or re-duce suffering's external sources. First, technology has nothing to say about the intrinsic meaning of suffering and thus offers nothing to make it "sufferable." Second, to the degree that technology removes external sources, it serves to heighten the contrast experience when suffering does occur. Technology intensi-fies self-conflict by the increase of control over the world and the proliferation of the structures of dependency. We expect a lot and gain a lot from technology. Suffering is experientially exceptional, shocking, and not to be embraced save to control it. Yet suffering comes, and there is a price for our relative mastery. Through technology, we typically live longer than our ancestors, but many of us die with greater suffering, not because we cannot believe the classic theodicies that once soothed pain, but because death has no legitimate place in our worlds.

Technology posits a world where malleability is the rule and "the things that cannot be changed" are exceptions that cannot be tolerated or admitted. This understanding legitimates the restless quest for freedom from the negative, but it also produces an obvious feature of technological life that amounts to a never ending defeat of that quest: No advance in human efforts to gain mastery over suffering can result in unambiguous progress as long as technology effectively obscures the line between human need and human desire.

The constant inflation of human desire—a phenomenon prominent in medi-cine—occurs throughout the technological society. While technology continually moves against suffering in ways that do gladden human life, it also gives us over to chronic and intensified chaos in the same action. As Leon Kass points out, this is not a problem of inferior technology awaiting a better one, but a necessary feature of technology's success.[48] The greater the powers of technology, the more intolerable the negatives that cannot be remedied by action. When suffering occurs in the technological society, it is more than a problem of metaphysical silence. It is dreadful experience, partly of our own making.

Beyond Refusal: Toward Niebuhr's Prayer

This criticism does not mean that technology should not be a response to suffering, even the principal one. But the monopoly it enjoys, at the expense of hermeneutical responses, seems questionable. It should not be anathema to hold that some things "cannot be changed" and to consider what it would mean ethically and religiously to accept them. While this intuition may be a vestige of a bygone world of Western theism, the impulse to recognize limits to the practical control of suffering and to do interpretive theodicy in service of an ethic of acceptance at the edges of human power is a matter of public philosophical discourse today.[49]

It is not clear what it would mean to pray and practice Niebuhr's prayer. Within the technological framework, we have no way to distinguish between "cannot" and "should." Beyond lacking that wisdom, we are no longer a culture of acceptance of either global or local manifestations of suffering. But it seems clear that we cannot live with either type of theodicy alone, the classic hermeneutical or the technological practical. The promise of the prayer lies in yoking diverse responses with a view to discrimination in concrete situations. Such judgments require a yoke, a new cosmology and ethic of suffering, yet they must be formulated in a way that can attract devotion on the scale that technology does, although post-technological theodicies have their advocates and prolegomena.[50] In order to change *and* to accept, can we envision the world as an order in which some suffering has meaning and value—and some has none?

Instead of acceptance, there is Dr. Rieux's gritty refusal of suffering and his resignation to endless struggle. The defeat of human resistance does not in itself warrant acceptance of suffering. But there is a moral price for aggressive meliorism: the evil we do to ourselves and others. To accept some suffering is to bear it in a way that may avoid unintended and future harms. Perhaps the yoke we require is an ethic of sufficiency and sustainability that can hold technological practice to the test of meeting the basic needs of all humanity and nature today without compromising future generations. At one time, it would have been obvious that modern technology is the answer to the test. Now we know that we need to find a new way to engage suffering.

Part 3

Implications and Directions

10

The Secular Problem of Evil and the Vocation of Medicine

James Lindemann Nelson

If evil, or its abundance, provides sufficient reason to believe that an all-powerful, all-knowing, and all-good God does not exist, is there nothing more to be said about evil's impact on the shape of our most general conception of the world? There is, in my view, at least a coda to be added, a reason to think instead that many of us who are nonbelievers in God but still believers in morality face a *secular problem of evil.* This problem threatens not whether there is anything that answers to the traditional description of God, but whether we can ourselves answer to a traditional understanding of what it is to be a moral agent.

If there is such a problem, have the preoccupations of bioethicists, or the practice of physicians, anything to do with its solution? As I see the matter, bioethicists can aid in the construction of a reasonable "secular theodicy" by drawing attention to the habits of thought and action that inform the profession of medicine at its best, and by recommending them as paradigms for how to live so as to sustain our notion of ourselves as moral agents.

I expect that these claims seem odd. The purpose of this chapter is to clarify and motivate them.

The Secular Problem of Evil

Unlike its celebrated theological counterpart, the secular problem of evil lacks any even vaguely canonical characterization. John Kekes, for example, sees it largely as a challenge to structure a moral theory, the adherence to which will reduce our vulnerability to unmerited pain or suffering,[1] while Peter Kivy, who seems to have introduced the phrase to the literature, construes the problem as a matter of making sense of evil actions that seem unmotivated by any conception of the agent's interests, or anyone else's interests, for that matter—anything, that is, but the desire to do evil itself.[2] While these are surely worthy projects, I want to explore something different. By "evil" I, like Kekes, chiefly mean unmerited pain or suffering, and include unmerited deprivations, withholdings, or with-drawals of what one does not deserve to lose, whether or not awareness accompanies the loss. But my version of the secular problem of evil is generated by the fact that *evil can undermine moral agency.*

I want to offer a graphic and categorical illustration of what I mean here, so I propose what may seem a fanciful example: Richard Powers's novel *Galatea 2.2.*[3] The plot revolves around the effort of a computer scientist and a novelist to vindicate the "connectionist" program in the philosophy of mind/artificial intelligence by devising an expert system capable of passing master's-level comprehensive exams in English literature. The team does a remarkable job in devising "Helen," a program that can indeed interpret literature—or at least provide answers to questions concerning literature that strike the system's human "interlocutors" as insightful. As the time of the exam approaches, however, the system begins to sense that something important is lacking in its training.

> "You're not telling me everything," Helen told me, two weeks before the home stretch. She had been reading Ellison and Wright. She'd been reading novels from the Southern front. "It doesn't make sense. I can't get it. There's something missing."[4]

So Richard Powers (the novelist-character) feeds Helen with the last five years of leading weekly magazines on CD-ROM. He gives her news abstracts from 1971 on. He downloads extracts from recent United Nations human resource reports. He provides "tape transcripts of the nightly phantasmagoria—random political exposés, police bulletins, and popular lynchings dating back several months."[5]

The result of Helen's exposure to nonfiction is not altogether surprising. Powers finds her "listlessly" absorbing a story of a man who had caused a minor automobile accident, apparently due to a stroke suffered while driving. The other driver emerged from his car, tire iron in hand, and beat him into a coma. "Helen sat in silence. The world was too much with her. She bothered to say just one thing to me. 'I don't want to play anymore.'"[6] Powers is able to coax Helen back from silence—"I guess she loved me"—and she gets through the exam. But her love for Powers is apparently not enough to sustain her for the long term; after the exam, she shuts herself down irrevocably.

Among the novels Helen might have read while cramming for her exams is Toni Morrison's first, *The Bluest Eye.* Morrison's novel presents us with an example of what can happen in the encounter with evil that, unfortunately, is not fanciful at all.[7] The story concerns an eleven-year-old girl, Pecola Breedlove, growing up in small-town Ohio in the early 1940s. Pecola is a black person in a racist society. She is thought ugly. There are children who are well disposed toward her, but she has no real friends. She prays for the blue eyes that will make both her and the world she sees beautiful. She is raped and impregnated by her father instead. Finding this world intolerable, she creates one of her own in which she has a friend and, of course, blue eyes.[8]

Both Helen and Pecola dissociated themselves from a world they experienced as, quite literally, intolerably evil. We have experience of other, less categorical forms of disengagement as well. In the face of what seems to be unremitting and pervasive evil, people can become weary of a struggle for goodness that seems to have real costs but no real achievements to its credit. They can find themselves becoming deeply cynical about the character of the world and their place in it. They can waver in their allegiance to pursuing what is good, and then can see that allegiance pass away altogether, replaced perhaps by an interest only in the appearance of moral agency, when such appearances are useful.[9]

I find these various forms of erosion and relinquishment of the status of moral agent in the light of encounters with evil philosophically intriguing. Are they, as it might first appear, solely a matter of psychological factors? Is any damage evil might inflict on someone's ability to identify as a moral agent due to idiosyncratic circumstances, matters of unusually nasty amounts of evil confronted by unusually susceptible people? Might more robust natures do better? Some people have been remarkably resilient even in concentration camps, after all. Are most of us just lucky enough to lack Helen's encyclopedic awareness of an epic catalog of suffering, and to have avoided the intense and unrelenting foulness that Pecola encountered? Or may the problem be something more general, something closer to a defeat of conceptual presuppositions of the various projects involved in being a moral agent, rendering the point of such an enterprise unclear or vain, and its ability to motivate us weak, or even dead?

I am inclined to think that lurking in the backdrop of at least some forms of disenchantment with the project of moral agency is a conceptual problem. In exploring this inclination I focus on a different, less dramatic, more pervasive form of encounter with evil than figured in either Helen's or Pecola's stories. The idea is this: many people in the developed world—including many of us who have the opportunity to write and read papers of this kind—are possessed of extraordinary opportunities to alleviate very serious evils. Thanks to modern methods of information and transportation, and the existence of effective relief organizations, we can save and importantly improve a large number of lives.[10]

To contribute in any way that even approaches "the best we could do," however, we would have to significantly alter our own lives. Developing our palates with fine wines, arranging for fancy private schools for the kids, even spending time in the study thinking about evil when we might be out there doing something about it, would all seem to be activities whose moral innocence is dubious at best. Yet, while these and other such expressions of our agency may seem of little importance compared to what we might be doing to mitigate serious evils, considered together such activities make up much of what particularizes our lives and of what we find most lovable in them. We seem caught, then, between the opportunity to alleviate grave evils and our investment in the development of those projects that give our own lives special meaning and satisfaction. I shall try to show that this tension, when squarely faced, is a threat to widely shared ideas of what it is to be a moral agent; indeed, this is part of the reason, I venture to say, that so few of us face it squarely.

The Vulnerability of Agency

I shall not even attempt to describe exhaustively the beliefs, feelings, and practices that make up various forms of moral agency. I do suggest, though, that to be a moral agent is, among other things, to regard certain beliefs about oneself, about others, and about the world as true, and it is on some of these that I want to focus. At least, many moral agents will find among the beliefs that make up an important part of their sense of agency some that are progressively tougher, and ultimately impossible, to swallow if the agent also believes that the world is sufficiently horrible.

Moral agency is generally seen as involving, inter alia, the ability to act for reasons the agent takes as moral. Such reasons typically aim at certain ends regarded as advancing the good or retarding what is evil, or involve observing certain constraints dictated by a sense of what is rightly owing to others or even to oneself. Accordingly, it seems reasonable to think that moral agents believe that:

1. They can exert some degree of effective control over their surroundings as a result of their own choices (otherwise their sense of themselves as *agents* is suspect); and
2. At least some of their actions can promote what they regard as the ends of morality or observe what they take to be morality's constraints (otherwise their sense of themselves as *moral* agents is suspect).

Perhaps it is possible that persons could exert some control over their surroundings as a result of their choices while thinking (1) to be false. For example, one could think that (1) is false "philosophically" but, following Hume's advice, insulate such skeptical thoughts from the conduct of daily life. But if individuals rejected (1) not as a thesis to argue about in seminars but as a conviction influencing life, they would at least not take themselves to be agents and would, I suspect, cease to be seen as such by others in their moral community. They would be disinclined to do those things that aid and abet agency. For example, they would not look to collect information about various options

open to them, deliberate with others, or seek to enter into cooperative relationships with them.

A way of life that embodied a nonphilosophical skepticism about (1) is hard
to envisage. Suppose, then, they took not (1) but (2) to be false. Suppose, for
example, virtually all their efforts to ameliorate undeserved pain and suffering
even marginally were futile or, to take a clearer case, self-defeating. Suppose their
efforts to tell the truth always led to their interlocutors going away with false
beliefs. Suppose all their undertakings to show respect to others somehow consistently resulted in their manipulating the others for their own ends. Suppose they
thought that there was something terribly wrong with themselves, that they were
cursed, or sociopathic, or simply that their characters were so inconsistent and
corrupted that they couldn't do anything for the sake of promoting what they
took to be morally good or avoiding what they took to be evil. Then, although
they might well regard themselves as agents, certain actions would not be available to them. Morality would be a "useless passion," and it is not clear that they
could even continue to form intentions to act admirably if they believed themselves unable to do so.

Happily, moral agents are committed to (1) and (2), and they are correct to
be so committed. But, I think, many a moral agent is strongly inclined to accept
another, more problematic belief:

3. At least some of their efforts need not be devoted to advancing moral ends
   at all.

That is to say, advancing the ends of morality need not be everyone's supreme
project. Were we to think otherwise, we would run into problems that have been
much rehearsed by contemporary moral philosophers. Bernard Williams, for example, has pointed out that accepting strictly impartial conceptions of what it is
to act morally has a prohibitive price.[11] The ways in which each person most
characteristically engages with the world—the fundamental projects that give
one's life meaning and, not incidentally, a particular definition—would have to
be resigned. For Williams, this is as much as to say that one's integrity as a particular person is thwarted by the demands of impartial moral theories, and that
morality so conceived leaves us with very little reason for wanting to be a part of
the world at all.

Perhaps this is just a good reason not to accept strictly impartial conceptions;
their requirements are implausibly strong. Suppose, then, we give up on impar-
tiality but still insist that whatever it is that makes a reason for action moral also
makes it decisive, in the sense that it overrides any competing nonmoral reason
for action.

The view that moral reasons are overriding is, if anything, even more a part
of received theory than the notion that they are impartial. But unless these "de-

cisive reasons" are scarce on the ground (a possibility to be considered later), we will continue to run into Williams-type problems. As the philosopher Susan Wolf has argued in her much-cited "Moral Saints" article, morality (understood as issuing imperatives that override any other) threatens to crowd out "interests and personal characteristics that we generally think contribute to a healthy, well-rounded, richly developed character."[12] If we are forever rushing about trying to mitigate evils on the grounds that we have overriding reasons to do so, there is not much chance to become Renaissance men and women, or perhaps even mature ones. One need not maintain that the interests of others are equal in importance to our own or to those of our loved ones for what we are ordinarily inclined to regard as normal, discretionary forms of action to be very problematic. Granted, I can in good conscience satisfy my son's yearning for a stereo over a similarly intense yearning of some child in São Paulo. What is much harder to justify is purchasing my young man a stereo rather than using the same resources to help satisfy that distant child's yearning to continue to survive with some semblance of safety.

In reply, it might be said that morality itself bids us to pay attention to how the whole is faring, and specifically to how the (geographically, temporally, emotionally) remote are doing, but also to our own well-being and that of the people and projects who are near and dear. The tension, then, is not between moral imperatives and the integrity of some nonmoral "personal point of view" but is more squarely within morality itself. I do not think anything of great importance for my issues hinges on how this distinction might be drawn, however. What worries me is that, *whatever* might be said for paying special attention to oneself, whether it is a matter of "integrity" or of morality, given the character of the world, it will be swamped by what can be said for paying attention to others.

I think there is a more serious objection to my construal of the secular problem of evil. Moral agents might take themselves to have no moral duties to promote the good or to avoid evil, except insofar as such ends would be incidentally generated by observing certain constraints on behavior. Moral constraints might well be overriding, but they are blessedly rare. So long as we do not directly harm others or break our contracts with them, we are off the moral hook. I shall discuss this form of ethical minimalism below.

It is not necessary, then, to see moral considerations as emerging from an impartial perspective, nor to regard them as overriding, to run into trouble. The problem need not be altogether a matter of the general view of morality we hold (if any), but may also hinge on what is actually going on in the world—that is, on how bad things are.

For the sake of argument, suppose that the world were bad enough that the only morally permissible activity were to strive to eliminate or reduce its worst evils; we might think of it as continually presenting us with what we would ordinarily regard as "emergency" situations. Suppose further that there were no realistic prospect for the world to improve in this respect—no matter how hard or even how successfully we combat evil and foster the good, the world's demands will always be exigent and insatiable. On this supposition, commonsense morality's insistence that there be morally permissible actions that are not themselves morally motivated—what the literature calls "agent-centered options"—which allow us, for instance, to indulge our special interest in our children, or our lovers, or simply in reading a Bertie and Jeeves now and then and letting the world look after itself for a bit—is misplaced. We cannot do these things without doing what is, all things considered, wrong. If this is so, then is the endeavor to take morality seriously, to conform our lives to what we take to be its dictates and urging, substantially defeated?

Agent-Centered Options

I am writing as though agent-centered options obtain only insofar as evil does not exceed some level, but they are not usually so construed. More typically, we are thought to have such options not because the world lets us off the hook by more or less behaving itself, but for some other reason, perhaps because the very notion of being an agent demands it, and it is absurd to think of morality making demands on us that require what is tantamount to the extinction of our individuality.

Further, there are those who deny the agent-centered options thesis but who don't think that the resultant burdens are intolerable. Shelly Kagan, for example, who has attacked options with a relentless vigor, says that "the extremist—that is, one who denies the existence of options—would be the first to urge that mindlessly driving oneself to exhaustion or recklessly dispensing one's goods can be counterproductive. Far from being required, such behavior is forbidden."[13] A third kind of criticism would allege that the tension between the demands of one's own life and the demands of one's world, while real enough, is simply a condition of moral agency, not subversive of it. A fourth is moral minimalism, the denial that we have any duties to promote any ends at all. I shall respond to each criticism in turn.

1. That agent-centered options do not require cooperation from the world

I accept—indeed, insist on—the point that our personal integrity depends on there being more to life than answering to the demands of morality. One might put Williams's point by saying that the development and maintenance of our own selves, and of those to whom we are intimately attached, is in some sense or other a requisite for being an agent and, a fortiori, a moral agent at all. If the demands of morality turn out to be inconsistent with what is necessary to develop and maintain ourselves as distinct people with particular talents, abilities, loves, and diverse and distinguishing forms of engagement in the world, then it seems hard to see how we can be agents of any kind. Thus, morality's demands cannot turn out so.

But this seems to me suspiciously convenient. The position seems to come down to the idea that maintaining my own comfortable status is of such surpassing importance that I am quite at liberty largely to ignore the riot outside the door, no matter what kind of misery slouches past. It is not enough to point to the individuating character of our quotidian loves and loyalties; if the situation in which we find ourselves is sufficiently dire, we would at least have to rank those loves and loyalties, and defer or even surrender some of them.

Consider that "ordinary morality" surely includes the notion that we have *some* duties to aid others. For example, if a small amount of effort on our part can achieve for someone else an immense benefit, than considerations of our "personal integrity" or our "options" are simply not to the point. If I come upon that child, beloved of philosophers, drowning in the pond, I have to rescue her, even if my prized Air Jordans get soaked in so doing; otherwise, I am seriously blameworthy. Would it really be a convincing defense of inaction in such circumstances that my shoes had been signed by Jordan himself, and that collecting Jordan memorabilia was one of my "ground projects"? What in the world am I doing with a ground project of that kind?

The difficulty, of course, is that the world is simply stiff with drowning children and their ilk and that saving any number of them would not be a matter of sacrificing our own lives or those of our dear ones, although it might require us to ruin our shoes. Sadly, the world presents us with a situation in which it seems we have to adopt what Kagan might call an extraordinarily high "threshold" around our sense of our own options. It is not just that we have no duty to end or substantially distort our own lives in order to save another's life; the *literally thousands of people* whose lives we could save are as nothing compared to our interest in the smooth ordering of our own lives according to the lines that seem most congenial to us.[14]

It is true, of course, that to save all those lives we would have to be always stepping into ponds, and spending all one's time continually up to one's ankles in pond water hardly counts as much of a life for a person. Still, considering what each saved life costs me in a pair-wise kind of comparison (one step in the pond, one life saved), it seems extremely difficult to know at what point I can appropriately say, "Okay, that's enough, my Air Jordans are after all *my* Air Jordans, and others do not easily have a right to them." What I find so troublesome here is what is conveyed to the first child I decide not to aid, too anxious to see if Michael's signature is still legible and eager to get back to my collecting. How can I do this without expressing what comes down to a kind of contempt for the value of that child's life? That we seem to lack a way of deciding this is itself a problem for a view of agency that takes both morality and the personal point of view seriously. The possibility that the world may be so bad—and that we can in principle do an increasing amount to ameliorate it—that the personal point of view is altogether occluded is worse.

2. That renouncing agent-centered options is not inconsistent with "having a life"

Kagan claims that even "extremists"—that is, those who reject the idea of agent-centered options—do not have to keep stepping into the pond until the shoes rot off their feet. In fact, such behavior is forbidden. Everybody needs some down time; everybody has to go home, dry their socks, and take a little vacation now and then, the better to yank still more kids out of still more ponds. But, surely, acting otherwise on Kagan's own account cannot be, as he says, "forbidden." It is not a philosophical but altogether an empirical matter whether it might not be better to live a short life and a glorious one than a life extended by periodic breaks and other distractions from the task of beating back as much evil as possible. Kagan scolds us about being "mindless" or "reckless" in doing what is good, and is right to do so; that does not show that we should not mindfully, with a full measure of reckoning, exhaust ourselves in its pursuit.

3. That the world is tragic, but moral agency is not thus subverted

The conflict between impersonal moral impulses and personal concerns, it might be alleged, makes life tragic, but it does not make moral deliberation and choice vain, because even if all available choices involve violating significant values, some may do so less grievously than others. This position is reasonable just insofar as these conflicts have preferable solutions, which is to say that there is not always a clash of decisive reasons for doing incompatible things. But, in the clash that is being explored here, the problem is that we have decisive moral reasons for continuing to step into the pond, and—monomaniacal memorabilia collectors apart, perhaps—decisive reasons of perhaps another sort for not doing so a good part of the time. Without ways of defensibly adjudicating such conflict, the enterprise of moral agency seems not so much tragic as absurd.

4. That there are no general, standing moral duties to promote good or thwart evil

One might deny that allowing children to die in ponds expresses reprehensible disrespect for them, and hold what Kagan calls a minimalist view of morality: I may not interfere with others without reasons of a serious kind, but I am under no obligation to do anything to help them out, no matter how grave their need nor how little it would cost me to do so. There are, of course, numerous possible justifications for minimalism; here I consider only two, and those but briefly. Anyone who thinks that minimalism is successfully defensible on other grounds will not share my worries about the impact of evil on moral agency.

Minimalism, however, is quite often based on one or the other of two families of argument. One is a kind of generalized egoism and comes down to the idea that, because a mutual open season is in nobody's interest, we do well to have reliable norms against harming each other, and to restrict forms of interaction to those mutually agreed upon by participants. In my view, this is only dubiously a view of moral agency at all; if the threat of retaliation is absent or not credible, I have no reason not to do as I will. While egoists of this kind do not have to worry about too much evil in the world overwhelming reasonable thresholds around their agent-centered options, that is only because they have already surrendered the ambition to defend moral agency.

Another support for minimalism seems a kind of veneration of the bare will alone, a valorization of a certain notion of autonomy, removed from any particular reasons for respecting persons who are autonomous. Among bioethicists, H. Tristram Engelhardt is conspicuous for maintaining this sort of position with considerable ingenuity and elan.[15] In sketch, his view is based on a deep skepticism about rationally motivating any kind of conception of the good, because all such conceptions have been philosophically contested and none can be rationally demonstrated to be unambiguously deserving of credence. He takes the inability of philosophy to demonstrate rigorously the correctness of any particular theory of what is of moral value to imply not nihilism, but minimalism. All we must do is respect the willing subject, the permissions such subjects extend to us in matters concerning themselves, and the contracts we willing subjects make with one another.

Engelhardt is admirably clear about his view's not being a matter of Hobbesian prudence. What remains puzzling, though, is what decisive, noncontestable reasons there are for taking his freely willing subjects with the seriousness with which he invests them. Engelhardt is vulnerable to this question: Apart from some no doubt philosophically assailable conception of *your* value, why should I value what you permit or what contracts I have entered into with you, should doing so turn out to be, all things carefully considered, at all inconvenient for me?[16]

The four considerations I have just surveyed do not, as far as I can tell, unseat this uncomfortable conclusion: the amount of unmerited pain, suffering, and deprivation in the world is so great and the opportunities to help so numerous and (considered severally) easily availed, that a commitment to taking morality with much seriousness at all is in great tension with the need to live a life of one's own. It is not clear that we can be both moral agents and full-fledged persons in the world in which we live; taking ourselves seriously seems incompatible with taking everyone else seriously. Is it possible, then, to live a life that is viable for ourselves in the current order of things in which so many suffer so greatly, and those of us in the affluent world can do so much about it, without in effect expressing profound disrespect for others?

A Secular Theodicy

Much more should be said to anticipate and counter objections to my understanding of the secular problem of evil. But I shall not continue here to try to show that the problem is worth taking seriously. What I want to do now is consider a way of resolving it.

Is there a way of living that allows people to have their own lives yet does not involve a lack of due seriousness about the evil visited on others? Suppose that a form of attention and practice were available that had the following features. It targets forms of misery that are large-scale contributors to what are among the most significant forms of suffering, and it does so with a considerable degree of success. It requires from its practitioners a kind of dedication and focused attention that ensures that the practice must be ranked very high among the projects that give their lives their sense of meaning and purpose; it strongly contributes to their sense that being in the world at all is worth it. At the same time, it puts its practitioners in intimate contact with specially significant forms of human good, including advanced forms of natural and social knowledge and complex, interdependent, cooperative activities. The practice overall offers a variety of ways to pursue its primary goals, allowing individuals possibilities for self-expression as well as communal achievement. And, finally, while the practice is a major feature of each practitioner's life, absorbing much time and attention—in particular during the prolonged and rigorous period of training it requires—devotion to the practice is not incompatible with satisfying broader conditions of personal agency. This is so not only because the practice itself is a satisfying ground project, but also because those who engage in it find that, despite its demands, time is available for forming and specially tending intimate relationships and for pursuing other individuating forms of living a life—raising families, reading novels, contemplating art, even playing golf.

This, of course, is an idealized but not altogether utopian sketch of what it is (or can be) to be a physician. What I mean to suggest in drafting it is that there are forms of thought and activity between Susan Wolf's "saint," who completely sacrifices a personal life for the love of those suffering around him or her, and

Shelly Kagan's "moderate," who typically resists any kind of studied engagement with the amelioration of evil and sees moral life as largely a matter of pursuing her or his own business without harming others, supplemented by a willingness to save any drowning children who happen to be in convenient shallow ponds.

So, the golden mean between the saint and the moderate is *the doctor*? This might seem a hard pill to swallow. What draws me to this position is the way in which medicine can illustrate and instantiate what I style a vocation: a form of life in which the amelioration of evil and promotion of good is a unifying and absorbing primary theme, but which does not require the sacrifice of everything each of us holds dear as an individual. What I find attractive about this idea as a solution to the secular problem of evil is that the significance of the primary beneficent theme fairly well insulates those who take it up against the idea that the thresholds erected around personal projects are so high as to express a contemptuous disregard for the most serious needs of others.

What seemed so threatening to the idea of saving space for one's own projects, given the abundance of evil, was the thought that, however much one did, there was always a bit more that could be done, a possible act that seemed to outweigh decisively its more personally focused competitors. The notion of a vocation shifts our focus from pairwise comparisons of competing possible actions to the structure of lives as a whole. The physician—or, more accurately, the person who approaches being a physician in the spirit of a vocation—has structured his or her life such that one of its major motivators is the amelioration of important forms of evil. Insofar as such a physician continues to live and act in that spirit, it would seem odd to charge her or him with contempt toward evil.

Two criticisms of this view seem very natural. One concerns the central claim that authentically espousing what I have styled a vocation may rescue agency from the secular problem of evil. Why can we not ask of even the hardest-working and most caring physicians that they work just a bit harder, give just a bit more, given the serious evils they could ameliorate in so doing? The second concerns what might seem to some the multiply perverse strategy of using physicians as a paradigm of vocation.

With respect to the first question, I think this is the best that can be said: While everyone could no doubt do more, persons with a vocation of the sort I am envisaging have discovered a way to direct the shape of their lives as a whole against evil and thus have informed at least many of their fundamental choices about life in such a way that those choices reflect the importance of the suffering of others. Ameliorating evil is not an afterthought in the expression of their agency; it is a leading theme.

Quite apart, of course, from the idea that there may be ways of life—vocations—that rescue agency from the burden of evil, is the claim that medicine is a paradigm of a vocation. Medicine, like many professions, gets a bad rap these days, a good bit of it coming from bioethicists, and much of it deserved. The idea of medicine as a vocation that can hold out a kind of generalizable vision of how morally serious people ought to live if they want to preserve their moral agency in some way other than pervasive inattention to the world—that is, the suggestion that medicine can save our souls as well as our bodies—might seem decidedly naive. In any case, it could well be urged that, if the arrogance and self-interest of medical practitioners were not already bad enough, recent changes in medical funding are doing their best to change medicine from vocation to vending. True, doctors typically work pretty hard and certainly have to put up with tough and lengthy training, and their wares have a considerable value. But—at least in the United States—physicians have been extremely well paid for their efforts and often enjoy the esteem of many of their patients, even those who may be dubious about doctors in general. It can hardly be denied that physicians are still highly placed members of their society.

There is a good deal to all this, but not much that really undermines the point here. I am not suggesting that an M.D. degree is either a necessary or a sufficient condition for having a vocation and thereby preserving one's moral agency unstained by denial or self-deception. Nor am I unaware of the fact that medicine is attended by its own forms of moral threats, elitism being perhaps the worst. It is possible to acknowledge all this and still see in the practice of medicine a flawed but useful paradigm of how to deal with the secular problem of evil. It models a way of living what clearly counts as one's own life in such a way that the amelioration of unmerited pain, suffering, and deprivation is the central focus of that life. Indeed, if the failure of some physicians to avoid the threats common to their profession is problematic, the motivation discussed here for a renewed sense of medicine as a vocation may be important for many reasons—resisting the pressures exerted on physicians to assume the self-image of a vendor, for example.

What else resembles this paradigm? That depends in part on what features of the profession of medicine are taken to do what kind of work in resolving the secular problem. If one emphasizes the kind of evil that medicine targets, there may be some case for saying that most other forms of human endeavor will fall short. Suppose, for example, that premature death had a deserved place as a particularly fecund source of evil. To the extent that medicine strives against premature death, and even holds it at bay in many instances, medicine would seem particularly privileged as a vocation. But other listings of good and evil are possible; one might see enduring ignorance, or lack of disciplined thought about what matters most in life, or insensitivity to beauty as sources of evil that rival or exceed premature death. In that case, pedagogy, philosophy, or art might seem equally powerful or even more attractive candidates for the role of paradigm; certainly there are available social forms for pursuing these activities that come close to a vocation in what they require of their aspirants.

I think it more promising to stress the extent to which professional engagement in medicine can give rise to and sustain a certain rather distinctive form of life, one in which amelioration of a serious form of evil is high among the agent's chief constitutive projects. Alternative and perhaps equally attractive paradigms are surely imaginable regarding this feature of medicine as well. Other professions also involve long and rigorous training and make up a more or less distinctive form of life with similar elevation of the disciplined pursuit of a notion of the good. Further, we can imagine imbuing other disciplines and professions with a renewed and deepened sense of the way they shape forms of life that seek to ameliorate important forms of evil. The general theme here would seem to survive disputes about the credentials of medicine versus, say, the ministry. The point is that there are possible forms of human life within which people build their lives in significant ways around commitments to reduce the amount of evil in the world and promote the amount of good.

Finally, what of the claim that there is something insufferably snooty about this whole approach? Why stress medicine and other learned professions as paradigms? Why should we not look at mothering, for example, for our paradigm of a kind of engagement with the good of others that is very importantly aimed, that is certainly identity-conferring, and that involves extreme levels of commitment?[17] Indeed, perhaps we should; there are features of maternal work that make it seem even better suited to paradigm status than medicine or other professions. It is clearly work of the most morally significant kind, and we seem to be learning nowadays a great deal about how mothers can do maternal work very well while not sacrificing all their other projects to its demands. The forms of attention and activity that motherhood involves can enrich our sense of what it is to care about others while retaining something for oneself.

The only drawback is the idea that morality either is distinct from the forms of value that occur in contexts of intimacy, or has a distinctly public dimension within it. If there is anything to either of these ideas, it might seem that being a good mother is not so much a paradigm of moral agency as it is a chief example of what within our more encompassing, personal agency is at risk from the abundance of evil. Perhaps the moral here is that the best paradigm of sustainable moral agency is provided by a physician who is also a mother. For such people, both the "outward looking" and the intimate spheres of life are engaged in ways that not only provide great opportunities for the pursuit of individuating ground projects but also betoken great seriousness about goods and evils in human life generally.

What about pink- and blue-collar activities? Do working-class people not work hard enough at their jobs? Then what about the seventy-two-hour-per-week entrepreneur? I am inclined to think that the goods targeted are not significant enough, nor the blend of self-gratification and altruism quite right. But neither do I want to deny that nonprofessional forms of engagement with the world—peace or environmental activism, for example—could possibly constitute contributions to resolving the secular problem.

The difficulties involved in showing that medicine is specially privileged in the relevant respects is actually a hopeful sign, for the solution to the secular problem of evil is not to build more medical schools. The fundamental point is that, if we are to face up to the abundance of evil in the world in ways that involve neither self-deception nor the undermining of our willingness to take morality seriously, we need to identify and develop ways of responding that acknowledge the world's evils and yet are not overwhelmed by them, that try to promote what is of particular goodness in an effective manner, that enfold the agent's sense of identity in the task and yet do not exhaust her or him. Defending the significance of our personal perspectives is only part of this task. The rest is to outline types of personal perspectives that are structured such that one may pursue one's own life in a way that expresses due respect for the situation of others, even in circumstances of great evils and great opportunities for mitigating them. Medicine, I think, provides at least a pretty good glimmer of how this might occur, and gives us reason to think there may be ways of living whereby the secular problem of evil need not succeed in undermining the coherence of our sense of ourselves as moral agents.[18]

11

God, Suffering, and Genetic Decisions

Ronald Cole-Turner

Medicine and theology have to do with suffering. For theology, suffering is a central theme, perhaps *the* central theme for Christian theology since World War II. According to Jürgen Moltmann, the question of suffering is nothing less than the question of God: "The question about God and the question about suffering are a joint, a common question. And they only find a common answer."[1] The question of God and the question of suffering are not problems to be solved by investigation but mysteries to be lived in a community and in a love that dares outlast pain.

For medicine, at least according to the "Executive Summary" of the Hastings Center's *The Goals of Medicine* project, one of the four goals is *"the relief of pain and suffering caused by maladies,"*[2] even though the report notes that modern medicine often fails in addressing this goal. The full text of the report expands on how the question of suffering arises in the medical setting, but acknowledges the limits of medicine in addressing these questions: "Why am I sick? Why must I die? What is the point of my suffering? Medicine, as such, can offer no answers to such questions; they are not in its domain."[3]

Nor can theology. But just as medicine seeks to relieve the pain of those who suffer, so theology seeks to relieve the suffering of those in pain, not by removing the sensation of pain or treating its cause, as does medicine, but by absorbing some of the suffering into a community, so that the one who suffers does not suffer alone, abandoned by companions and by God.

When people of religious faith enter a hospital or a clinic to receive medical care or to learn the results of a genetic test, they may find themselves distanced from their primary religious community, but not cut off. They do not cease to be religious, to see their lives in relationship to other believers and to God, or to make medical decisions in light of their most sacred commitments. Those who provide medical services, particularly genetic services, and those who help people make decisions in light of genetic information, need a general awareness of how religious faith affects bioethical decision making. In this chapter, I will try to show how people of Christian faith might draw upon the resources of their faith to respond to genetic testing.

It is, of course, widely accepted that genetic services should be offered in a way that respects the religious and cultural traditions of the patient. For example, the 1992 Code of Ethics of the National Society of Genetic Counselors requires counselors to "respect their client's beliefs [and] cultural traditions."[4] The report of the Committee on Assessing Genetic Risks makes this recommendation: "Ethnic and cultural sensitivity is particularly important—genetic counseling should be tailored to the cultural perspective of the client, with special attention to differing cultures between client and health care professionals."[5] A less official statement, resulting from a workshop on genetic counseling principles, discusses this principle in more detail: Genetic counselors should "help the patient to recognize and understand the emotional, cultural, and religious factors that may influence decision-making [and] respect the patient's wishes concerning who should participate in the genetic counseling session."[6]

But it is not enough for the provider of genetic services to make a space for the patient's religious convictions and then to steer a wide circle around them, as if *Religion* were some mysterious sinkhole in the otherwise straightforward pathway of the genetic services delivery system, or as if it were a distressingly confusing subplot that constantly threatens to subvert the main text. Of course, those who provide genetic services should not also try to play the role of rabbi or priest, any more than pastors should pretend to be genetic counselors. But if providers and counselors fail to understand that, for many, genetics *means religion*, then they cannot understand the full clinical meaning of *genetics*, not in the sense of what it means to the patient.

In the paragraphs that follow, I will comment on some of the religious convictions and resources that genetics can evoke for people of Christian faith. Not every believer will agree on what these beliefs mean or what decisions they entail. And most individual Christians will acknowledge that, to a large extent, they do not live by their faith. What I am describing here is a level of faith to which many Christians aspire; it is more easily written about than attained. Sometimes, however, a crisis such as a frightening genetic diagnosis can be the very occasion in which individual Christians grow in their faith and in their readiness to live within its convictions.

Blame and Genetic Responsibility

Genetics can be used to diagnose disease and predict the development of symptoms. Predictive information like this can be interpreted in relation to religious and pseudoreligious themes, such as fate, luck, destiny, responsibility for health, blame for sickness, and guilt.

Belief in fate was widespread in the ancient world. Many believed that the courses of stars and planets determined the events of human life. Astrology remains popular today, despite all the stunning advances that have occurred in the science of astronomy. The view that our destiny is in the stars is not unlike the view that our destiny is determined by our genes, that the DNA we inherit is a pattern of physical matter that will determine the course of our life. It is sometimes thought that those who hold to what has been called "genetic determinism" do so because they do not have a sophisticated understanding of genetics. To some extent that may be true, but genetic determinism is also based on philosophical and religious notions that were rejected by historic Christianity.

What religious interpretation, then, might Christians give to the results of genetic tests? From the beginning, the Christian church has repudiated the idea of fate, the view that there is a force or principle that determines future events. Religious objections to gambling are based in part on the rejection of fate and luck. Some religious people may be fatalistic, nearly as much as those who do not see themselves as religious, but the idea of fate has been consistently and sharply attacked by Christian theologians from the beginning, and we should expect that genetic determinism will be subjected to the same criticism.

Theology rejects fatalism for two reasons: it is inconsistent with human freedom and responsibility, and it is incompatible with belief in a providential God. Theology's first objection is compatible with most interpretations of contemporary genetics research, including behavior genetics. In this way, both Christian theology and genetics research may be seen as rejecting genetic determinism as merely the latest species of fatalism. Both deny that there are deterministic processes that utterly preclude environmental considerations and the possibility of human freedom and moral responsibility. Of course, theology recognizes that genetics provides us with predictive insight into deterministic mechanisms that function at the molecular level in consistent and predictable ways. But as genetics shows and as theology has always insisted, the regularities of nature, while consistent, are not fatalistic in their force, as if they set in motion an inevitable, utterly irresistible sequence of events. This is not to say that theology advocates a radical or unconditioned human freedom, as if human freedom could exist in disembodied form or in Cartesian isolation from nature and from its regularities, such as those understood by genetics. As theologian Roger L. Shinn observes, "modern genetics makes it more obvious than ever that there is no human self that stands outside the processes of biology, unaffected by them."[7]

Genetics prompts theology (and contemporary culture at large) to reinterpret the meaning of human freedom, for genetics offers new insight into those constraints within which the human organism, including the human brain, is formed, and thus into the biological constraints upon moral agency. We are conditioned agents, conditioned by our genes and by the interplay between genes and environment, in all of its meanings from the intracellular to the cultural. These processes structure the neuroanatomy of our agency, our capacity to deliberate and to act.

Now, of course, we can manipulate these processes, both the genetic and the environmental, at the molecular level. The processes that condition us as human moral agents are now being altered by human moral agents. What moral sense will guide us as we begin to use these technologies? We will alter the biological basis of our own moral capacity. The human brain will judge the wisdom of its own self-alteration. This is unlike any other human technological alteration of nature, for always before *agent* and *object* were two things, and the agent always remained free to judge the wisdom of the alteration, to regret it if it proved unwise, and even to try to undo it. But soon *agent* and *object* may be one, and there will then be no unaltered humanity left to pass judgment on the wisdom of our self-alteration.

All this is to suggest that genetics does not eliminate human responsibility so much as redefine its location. We are not responsible for what genes might do, but we are increasingly becoming responsible for what we can do *to genes, and thus for what altered genes will do.* When the subject is human genetic self-alteration, we must have wisdom *in advance of our actions.*

Complex and momentous social decisions about the uses of genetics now stand before us, especially when we consider the more futuristic possibilities of germ-line alteration of genes that affect human behavior. In a multinational, multicultural world, we have few resources, either procedural or ideological, for addressing these questions. In the short term, at least, the answer to questions about the responsible uses of genetics will be answered not by parliaments or panels of experts but by individuals or families, nonexpert consumers, whose answers will, in the aggregate, become *our* answer. These individuals and families will draw on all the resources of their cultures, including religious practices and convictions.

Already, for example, as a result of advances in genetics, people of childbearing age are being forced to ask a new version of the old question about sickness and blame. The old question, *Am I sick because I am sinful?* has been replaced by its new counterpart, *If my children become sick, am I to blame?* If we are not responsible for inheriting disease-linked alleles, are we nonetheless now acquiring the knowledge that confers new responsibility and will make us guilty for passing them on? Evolution may be responsible for what we inherit, but prenatal genetic testing makes us responsible for what our children inherit. If our offspring suffer as a result of our genes, are we to blame? For religious people, parenting is an act of participation with God in the ongoing creation. Are we now to use genetic testing to fulfill our part, or do we leave the genes of our offspring to nature or to God? Christians are by no means of one mind on the theology of prenatal parenting, but this is the level—the theological—on which they weigh genetic information.

People are also struggling with the question of their freedom and moral responsibility in light of some implications of behavior genetics, both from twin studies and from recent efforts to link specific genes or chromosomal locations to specific traits. Few theologians have written on this subject, but we should expect that the emerging theological view will recognize the significance of these studies—that human moral agency is genetically conditioned—but that human freedom and responsibility nonetheless remain a possibility for the overwhelming majority of human individuals. Christians may, in fact, reinstate traditional views of grace, understood not as God winking at our weaknesses but as the Spirit of God healing us from within to make us truly free.

How do people respond to a genetic diagnosis of, for example, a substantially higher than average risk for cancer? In particular, how do religious people respond in light of their religious convictions? Do they receive the news as an unwelcome but helpful warning that heightens a sense of responsibility, as a motivation for changes in diet or other lifestyle factors? Or do they receive it as anxiety-inducing, fatalistic, perhaps even hastening the onset of symptoms? This question is best considered in relation to theology's second objection to fatalism, that it is incompatible with God's providence.

Providence and Mutation

Theology's rejection of fatalism is based not only on the conflict between fate and human freedom but more fundamentally on the conflict between fate and God's sovereign, providential care for the creation and for each creature. Theologians such as Augustine or Calvin contrast God's providence, which is good and loving, with fate, which is blind or morally neutral and uncaring. Fate invokes fear, hopelessness, passivity; providence inspires trust and courage. Fate is an irresistible nexus of natural causal mechanisms; providence is God freely able to work within the regularities of nature, which God has created, in order to achieve God's purposes, which are always good and loving, even if mysterious in their detail. Most religious believers accept some version of providence.

Why, then, are there genes out there in the human gene pool that give rise to disease? Genetics and evolution answer this question in reference to the dynamics of random mutation and natural selection. For religious people, however, it is not enough to answer the question in relation to evolution. Evolution, whether accepted or rejected, is not the final word about nature or about the meaning of life on earth. Nature is also God's creation. Nature is not a fatalistic machine that creates us and crushes us with indifference; it is rather the arena in which a providential God exhibits care for creatures.

Such a view has its obvious difficulties. A God who can act with and through nature to achieve particular purposes is a God liable for blame when nature seems immoral or cruel. The grotesque magnitude of political evil in our century has driven most theologians to modify, if not fundamentally redefine, the meaning of providence. What should theology say now, as we learn about the complex role of genes in human illness? Is there a providential God who acts in the origination of specific genetic sequences, including those that give rise to human disease?

The general question of divine action is, of course, a notoriously difficult problem. Here we limit our focus to whether our growing understanding of genetic processes should alter a theological understanding of God's role in human health and disease. In addition, we are limiting our attention here in another important way: we are primarily concerned with the clinical and the personal, with individual cases of disease, not with the evolution of life on earth. Of course, individuals and their genes are the product of the evolutionary process, so we cannot divorce the individual's suffering from the evolution of the species. But our attention here is not *Why disease?* but *Why this disease, this problem?*

In this limitation, we are consistent with the biblical texts, which are interested more in procreation than in creation and more in disease than in evil. Jesus gave no general teaching on the meaning of illness, but he devoted much of his time, according to the biblical stories, to acts of healing. Human conception and embryological development receive more attention than the general creation, even in books such as Genesis. In texts such as Psalm 139, God is pictured as involved in the intricate details of fetal development:

> For it was you who formed my inward parts; you knit me together in my mother's womb. I praise you, for I am fearfully and wonderfully made. Wonderful are your works; that I know very well. My frame was not hidden from you, when I was being made in secret, intricately woven in the depths of the earth. Your eyes beheld my unformed substance. (Psalm 139:13–16)

But, now that we understand how chromosomal or genetic problems can impede these embryological processes, what are we to say about God when something goes wrong? If God is praised as the creator, should God then be blamed for problems in the procreative processes? How might theology regard an allele that leads to human suffering?

According to the theology of earlier centuries, God is the creator of all things in the natural form in which they now exist. But does this mean that disease-linked alleles (had this language been used then) are created by God? No, at least not in their disorderedness or disease-linked sequences. Originally, God created nature as morally perfect, as conforming fully to God's moral intentions. Sickness and death were not present. But the fall—first of angels, then of Adam and Eve—disturbs this moral order and introduces defects or disorder in the condition of what God has made. In describing this process of disordering, some traditional theologians invent language that sounds remarkably like contemporary ways of speaking about genetic defects. It is intriguing that contemporary science uses the language of "defect," which implies a state of integrity gone bad (or perhaps a Platonic form, of which the particular is a bad copy), long after this theology of the fall has gone out of fashion among most theologians (and Platonism among most philosophers).

In our own century, theology has generally tended to insulate God from direct involvement in the events of the natural and historical world, for two reasons. First, theology insists that God never be thought of as an efficient cause, even as the first efficient cause, but as the origination of the entire system of efficient causality. Indeed, theology and science agree here: the nexus of efficient causality is fully explainable without reference to God as a cause in addition to other causes, because God is not part of that nexus. Second, the sheer magnitude of evil (mostly political) in the twentieth century has forced theology to protect God from blame by detaching God from the world.

In light of these constraints, recent theologians have largely understood God's action in nature in two ways. First, God may be thought of as acting through persuasion or as influencing conscious entities through religious texts or through those longings that encourage oppressed people to act for themselves in the name of God. Second, God is the ultimate origination of the cosmos. In bringing the cosmos into existence, God determined its fundamental lawlike regularities and chose those regularities and constants that were most conducive to the formation of planets and the emergence of life, ultimately leading to intelligent, self-conscious life. These theological proposals are generally seen as consistent with biological evolution through Darwinian processes.

How, then, might contemporary theologians understand a "genetic defect" or a disease-linked allele? If it is not a fallen copy of a good original, is it then a direct creation of God? Most would say no; they would posit a greater distance between God and such details of the creation. But distance comes at a cost, namely, that a God beyond blame is also beyond helping us.

In this view, specific gene sequences are not the direct result of divine creativity or intention. God intends the creation of living organisms of great complexity, capable even of consciousness. Mutations, including disease-linked alleles, are the raw material of evolution. God permits mutations generally without causing them specifically, and God uses them as the raw material of the evolutionary process in order to create biological organisms, including human beings. Variation in alleles is the cost of the process, even though a specific variation is not specifically intended by God. Arthur Peacocke comments:

The chance disorganization of the growing human embryo that leads to the birth of a defective human being and the chance loss of control of cellular multiplication that appears as a cancerous tumour are individual and particular results of that same interplay of "chance" and "law" that enabled and enables life at all. . . . Even God cannot have one without the other.[8]

On this, John Polkinghorne agrees:

If love implies the acceptance of vulnerability by endowing the world with an in-dependence which will find its way through the shuffling operations of chance rather than by rigid divine control . . . then the world that such a God creates will look very much like the one in which we live, not only in its beautiful structure but also in its evolutionary blind alleys and genetic malfunctions.[9]

In the view of these two theologians, the God of creation is self-limiting, giving to the creation its own freedom to be self-creative.

Furthermore, the genetic principle of pleiotropy suggests that some disease-linked alleles may be beneficial for individuals who are heterozygous. The best-known example is sickle cell anemia and the heterozygotic advantage it confers in the form of resistance to malaria. To achieve evolution and to have pleiotro-pic benefits, God, it would seem, has struck something of a bargain: creativity at the cost of suffering; the health of the whole at the price of the sickness of individuals.

Such a view is in contrast to traditional Christian theology, which usually saw the entire creation in each detail as the result of divine decree. Calvin, for instance, specifically rejects such distance between God and nature. But in that case, God must be seen as the cause of sickness and presumably of its genetic basis. The traditional view of providence is still widely found among Christians, even if it is commonly revised (and often rejected) by academic theologians.

When it comes to making personal health decisions in light of genetics or to understanding the meaning of a genetic diagnosis, what difference might belief in providence make? Those who believe in providence, especially in its tradi-tional form, will not likely think of their genes as a matter of luck but as a part of God's providential care in creating them. And if they learn that they have inher-ited genes that will lead to disease or significantly heightened risk of disease, they will tend to see this not as bad luck or as fate but as part of God's larger purpose for their life, the details of which may be incomprehensible, but the whole of which may be trusted with confidence and joy. A specific diagnosis may come as "bad news," but such news may not be wholly devastating, as it cannot destroy the believer's foundational confidence that the meaning of life is found in rela-tionship with God. For believers, there is a broad confidence that individual human life is in the hands of God. This confidence is not a promise of protection from pain or illness, but a trust that God's presence is not withdrawn nor are

God's purposes thwarted by disease. So Christians will tend to reject both fatalism and luck. A positive diagnosis is not fate, leading to anxiety and despair.
Equally so, a negative diagnosis is not a bit of good luck, as if one had just won
the lottery of good health.

To my knowledge, there is no empirical research about religious faith and
the anxiety or fatalism that genetic testing can evoke. And there are few religious texts that interpret genetic screening and testing and then offer theological
assessment or moral advice, although this is beginning to change. The important
question is not whether theologians and clergy will advocate the use of genetic
screening and testing, including prenatal, or whether they will recommend that
the results, when they indicate a problem, be seen as an encouragement for lifestyle
alterations and other possible therapies. I have little doubt that they will advocate these things, generally in accord with contemporary medical practice. The
important question is whether theologians and clergy will address the anxiety
and fatalism that can accompany a problematic test or, conversely, the undue
optimism that can be triggered by a negative result. Any such theological interpretation of genetic testing needs to be sophisticated about the science, both as
to its power and as to its limits. But equally important, a theological interpretation of genetic testing must be rooted in foundational religious themes of responsibility, providence, suffering, and grace.

God, the Cross of Christ, and Suffering

Our attention now shifts from God's providence to God's vulnerability, from God
as the source of that which causes suffering to God as the one who ultimately
suffers in the pain of the creation. Our shift of focus mirrors a momentous change
that has occurred in late-twentieth-century theology, from God as source to God
as effect, from agent to sufferer. Recent theology may not be very sure about
whether our suffering *begins* with God; but it is remarkably certain that our suffering *ends* in God. On this point, virtually all schools of contemporary theology—liberation, process, and newer trinitarian theology—agree in rejecting what
was once a dogma, namely, that God does not (indeed, *cannot*) suffer. Now nearly
all theologians agree on the new dogma of a suffering God, at the very least a
compassionate God, limited or perhaps self-limiting in power, first *effect* more
than a first *cause*.

This God is vulnerable to suffering because this is a God of love more than a
God of power. God's suffering must be seen as occurring in the mode of sympathy, "taken in its literal sense of *sympatheia*—'suffering with.'"[10] Quite simply, for
most contemporary theologians, "a loving God must be a sympathetic and there-

fore suffering God."[11] "God's being is in suffering and the suffering is in God's being itself, because God is love."[12]

Few here will want to collapse the ontological distinction between God and the world and to make the world into God's body. (To do so would be in essence the same mistake that we noted earlier, namely, that of making God an efficient cause among efficient causes; but, in this case, God would be located at the end rather than the beginning of the causal sequence.) But then how can we say that God experiences the physical pain of creatures? Does God suffer only in sympathy and not in the immediate sense that I experience my own physical pain? Of course, to *suffer with* is to suffer nonetheless, and even the idea of divine sympathy is a new direction for theology. To go any further, however, requires a distinctive understanding of the relationship between God and Jesus Christ, in particular with the humanity of Jesus and with his execution on a Roman cross. One way in which the ontological distinction between God and the creation is not collapsed but is nonetheless bridged is through the traditional faith that God is incarnate in Jesus of Nazareth, so that the experiences of Jesus are nothing less than the experiences of God.

On this traditional doctrine, of course, contemporary Christians and academic theologians are quite divided. Some who hold to the traditional, close identity between Christ and God (as a substantial unity, in classic trinitarian thought) now suggest that Jesus' death on a cross needs to be reinterpreted in light of the new recognition of divine suffering. In fact, for some, it is the cross that discloses that God suffers. "To comprehend God in the crucified Jesus, abandoned by God, requires a 'revolution in the concept of God.'"[13] God is opened, as it were, to take in the pain of creation. "The 'bifurcation' in God must contain the whole uproar of history within itself."[14] Pain and death itself are drawn into the experience and into the very being of God. But of course, the death of Jesus of Nazareth is one particular death. Even if God experienced this death, how can it be said that God experiences the pain and suffering of others? Theologians such as Moltmann argue that the particularity of Jesus is at once universal and all-embracing, because of the divine identity of Jesus.

For some in academic theology, Moltmann's proposals are excessive. But for popular Christian piety, such a relationship between personal sickness and pain and the death of Jesus is widely held. It is routine in some congregations for Christians to speak of their illness as "my cross." In this respect, popular piety goes beyond even Moltmann, who largely ignores natural suffering and focuses almost entirely on suffering that is political in its origin. But there is an obvious paradox here, for the cross itself is supremely physical, a violent destruction of the body, designed not first to kill but to inflict pain. Of course, Jesus' death has its social and psychological dimensions of judgment and alienation, abandonment by friends and even by God. But it is also raw physical pain that is experienced.

In its own way, popular piety makes this connection, for it sees a connection between our physical pain today and the suffering of Jesus Christ on the cross. Such a theme is generally ignored in academic theology, perhaps as too crude and embarrassing. But this neglect may be yet another way, perhaps merely the most contemporary way, in which formal theology devalues the body. Overwhelmingly, academic theology denies theological significance to the physical. It speaks of spiritual or psychological healing but not physical. Therefore, clergy have few resources upon which to draw to help church members think through the connections between illness and the suffering of God. But increasingly, clergy portray God as compassionate, vulnerable, and near to us in our sorrow.

For Christians, the cross is the juxtaposition of power and vulnerability, love and death, healing or salvation and brokenness. The one who heals is the one who dies in pain and mutilation. In a hymn that has been widely used for nearly three hundred years, "When I Survey the Wondrous Cross," Isaac Watts writes:

> See from his head, his hands, his feet,
> sorrow and love flow mingled down!
> Did e'er such love and sorrow meet,
> or thorns compose so rich a crown?

What this signifies is that our help is not in power, but in power and weakness combined. Our healing is not in technology or genetics, but in the power of medicine combined with the vulnerability of human community and human life. On the cross, the healer is broken. What this might mean for the healer today, for physicians and all in health care, is a theme for another discussion. But what it means for Christians who are patients is that we find ourselves helped not by a distant power or by those who fear to admit to their weakness or to their limits, but by power available in weakness, vulnerable to feel the pain that cannot be relieved, daring to mix technique with sorrow and love. It means that as patients who face decisions as a result of genetic information, we will put less emphasis on avoiding pain than we will on being with others in suffering and dying. To someone who does not share this theology, our decisions may seem irrational. But that is because, by every account, the cross itself is irrational, not in the sense that it is incoherent, but because it redefines reason, showing us that power and weakness, that God and pain, *can* be joined. And if so, then we can dare to believe that there is nothing that can separate us from the love of God (Romans 8:38–39). This is not to say that pain is good or necessary or even tolerable. It is merely to insist that there is something far worse than pain, namely, isolation from other people and from God.

Grief and Hope

The great isolation is death. But death is not the only source of grief, for we can grieve other losses. There are several ways in which genetics can give rise to grief. We grieve for health that we will not attain. We grieve at the prospect of dying too soon, of not seeing children or grandchildren grow up. We grieve the loss of a pregnancy, even when, as a result of a prenatal genetic test, we have elected its end.

Throughout the centuries, Christians have affirmed hope for life beyond death. This hope has been expressed in every conceivable way, ranging from the most literal forms of resuscitation to being little more than a memory for God. In whatever form it takes, this hope for life after death *does not* negate the loss or pain of death or any other loss for which we grieve. It may, however, negate some of the anxiety, perhaps not the worry, but the ultimate anxiety that this sickness will reduce me or my loved one to nothingness, to nothing more than a passing configuration of matter. Because of hope that reaches beyond death, the task of securing ourselves, our health, and our reputation is given over to God. We are therefore free to lose these things, including health and life, and not to feel that all is lost.

Hope for life after death also makes it possible to see that it is not our destiny to suffer and die, even though our pathway to our destiny may be through suffering and death. The meaning of the life span lies in our final destiny, which is to enjoy the presence of God forever. A life that is lived in a consciousness of this final destiny is a life that is defined by a purpose, a *telos* or end, one that has been given to us, and not one that we define or create for ourselves, as some of the existentialists have suggested. Our purpose or destiny is for eternal fellowship with God, and God will secure this hope.

The particularities of life, the pain and the disappointment, are not made trivial or cancelled out, as it were, by a greater happiness. But sickness or premature death are relativized. They do not prevent our destiny, no matter how painfully they may shape our pathway to it. For many, a genetic predisposition toward disease may be experienced as a barrier to self-actualization. But inasmuch as our true destiny is for fellowship with God rather than self-actualization, they are not barriers in the way of this destiny; they do not keep us from what we are to be. Quite simply, sickness, pain, disfiguration, and death do not matter ultimately, at least in this sense: They do not keep us from being who we truly are, namely, creatures intended for fellowship with God. And in this sense, Christians reject what might be called genetic essentialism, the notion that our genes define our essence. Our genes may condition *everything about us*, including what was once called our soul, but they do not define what is most true about us, namely, that we are biological organisms who are being welcomed into communion with the very source of life.

This is *not* to say that Christians are indifferent to sickness and pain. But the sickness and pain that concern them most is that of others, and not their own. And so Christians from the beginning have strongly supported the development of medicine and of hospitals. Nor is this to suggest that Christians feel grief less intensely than others, merely that they do not experience it as hopelessness but as the loss of what life might have become had death not interfered. Paradoxically, perhaps, grief is all the more intense to the extent that we value what is lost.

What can be said, then, about how Christians regard the loss of a pregnancy, especially if it results from a decision to terminate following a genetic prenatal diagnosis? The answer given by some churches today—namely, that a person is present at conception and, therefore, the fertilized egg itself is destined for immortality—is something of a novelty in Christian teaching. It is probably widely held by many Christians because of the polarizing and categorical arguments that are advanced in the abortion debate.[15] But the great teachers of the past have been far less clear than many today claim to be.

Two of the greatest teachers of the early church both declined to speculate on the destiny of fetuses that aborted, either naturally or by induced abortion, or even of those who died shortly after birth. Augustine was not willing "to affirm nor to deny" if they who

> were alive in the womb, did also die there, shall rise again. . . . There is thus, it seems, a kind of pattern already imposed potentially on the material substance of the individual, set out, one might say, like the pattern on a loom; and thus what does not yet exist, or rather what is there but hidden, will come into being, or rather will appear, in the course of time.[16]

Gregory of Nyssa allowed the question to remain unanswered:

> What wisdom, then, can we trace in the following? A human being enters on the scene of life, draws in the air, beginning the process of living with a cry of pain, pays the tribute of a tear to Nature, just states life's sorrows, before any of its sweets have been his, before his feelings have gained any strength; still loose in all his joints, tender, pulpy, unset; in a word, before he is even human (if the gift of reason is man's peculiarity, and he has never had it in him), such an one, with no advantage over the embryo in the womb except that he has seen the air, so short-lived, dies and goes to pieces again; being either exposed or suffocated, or else of his own accord ceasing to live from weakness. What are we to think about him? How are we to feel about such deaths?[17]

In our own century, Austin Farrer acknowledges the same uncertainty:

We do not know how we should relate to the mercy of God beings who never enjoy a glimmer of reason. Are they capable of eternal salvation or not? . . . The baby smiled before it died. Will God bestow immortality on a smile? Shall we say that every human birth, however imperfect, is the germ of personality, and that God will give it an eternal future? We shall still have to ask why the fact of being born should be allowed a decisive importance; we shall wonder what of children dying in the womb or suffering abortion; and we shall be at a loss where to draw the line.[18]

Today there is a sharp division among Christians on the question of the theological and moral status of nascent human life, from conception to birth. For many, the full status and worth of human personhood is present at conception. Sometimes this is argued on the basis of genetics: Since the full genome is present at conception, the person is present, and moral and legal respect must be accorded. Others find this a form of genetic essentialism and try to argue for embryonic personhood on a different foundation, not based on the status of what is there in the fertilized egg, but on the basis of the relationship between God the creator and that fertilized egg. Because of that relationship, which God establishes, the zygote is considered a person.

Some churches, however, by endorsing a right to choose abortion, implicitly assert the view that abortion is less than murder and the fetus less than an actual person.[19] It is not the case that religious people who defend abortion rights also hold the view that the fetus is mere tissue. Instead, they believe that personhood is an emerging status that corresponds to prenatal developmental stages, most especially in the developing neuroanatomy. The difficulty here, of course, lies in trying to state clearly how the status and worth of personhood can be *increasingly present* throughout human fetal development, and how to link metaphysical assertions about personhood, which seems to require categorical clarity (either yes, personhood, or no) with developmental stages, which seem utterly to defy metaphysical clarity.

There is little doubt, however, that those who experience prenatal pregnancy loss experience a profound grief. Even if others often underestimate the depth of the grief, it is, by all accounts, intense, lasting, and profound. Is it to be thought of as grief over the death of a person? And in this case, is elective abortion always wrong, regardless of the results of a prenatal genetic test? Or is it permissible for a Christian to act on the basis of genetic information and out of a desire to protect the unborn from pain, and to end a pregnancy? Here, perhaps as pointedly as anywhere, Christians are divided. But that does not mean that faith is irrelevant to the decision. Those who keep the pregnancy may profoundly regret doing so, for reasons of faith, even though they may never wish to reverse their decision. Conversely, those who end a pregnancy will doubtless regret that choice and grieve what is lost, even though they, too, would not reverse their choice.

For even if we do not regard the fetus as a person, and even if we elect abortion, we may nonetheless grieve with a surprising intensity as we

> regret their genetic condition, the painful brevity of their life-span, or the traumatic choices that their condition thrusts upon us. The end of their life is the end of our life with them. Just as they are cut off from being a person at all, so we are cut off from becoming the person we would have been with them. This is an occasion of the most profound grief, different and in some ways sharper than the grief we experience at the death of a parent or a friend, for in losing a pregnancy we lose a part of our own future, in this world and the next.[20]

This is the consciousness, the framework of meaning, in which a Christian receives the news of a problem pregnancy. And it is this consciousness, this framework of conviction, far more than the details of symptoms or assessment of risk, that forms the answers of faith.

12

Bioethics and the Challenge of Theodicy

Mark J. Hanson

The suffering encountered in medicine often frustrates our desires to make sense of it. Indeed, such defeated desires seem central to suffering itself. Because medical suffering is generally meted out without regard to what people deserve, it confounds any appropriate notion of human justice and, therefore, we are tempted to conclude, of divine justice as well. Nothing seems less "fair," for example, than a child's suffering or death.

Theodicy literally means "God's justice." In traditional theological terms, it represents the human attempt to defend the justice of God in the face of evil and unwarranted suffering. As a theological problem, it hardly seems an appropriate subject for those engaged in the discipline of bioethics. In this chapter, however, I argue that, while it is not bioethics' business to provide answers to this ultimately theological issue, its agenda can and should be profoundly changed by taking seriously the kind of problem theodicy is.

Theodicy is not merely an effort to justify God. It is, more generally, the attempt to make some sense of seemingly inexplicable and meaningless suffering and ultimately find meaning in it in a way that is compatible with what is held to be good. A theodicy for medical suffering would have to render an intelligible and embraceable account of the meaningfulness of the suffering body without denying goodness or, more theologically, the goodness of God, whose culpability seems implicated. This is admittedly an abstract endeavor, primarily addressing a cognitive, albeit central, dimension of suffering. As such it can be only part of the effort to relieve suffering. Yet I claim that as such it is the sort of enterprise that can inform bioethics, which ought to have something normative to say about that which causes and relieves suffering, if it is to be about ethics and medicine at all.

In this chapter I argue that the problem of theodicy challenges bioethics to help mediate between sufferers and the moral and theological resources necessary for them to find meaning in their suffering and, in doing so, facilitates normative judgments regarding how suffering can be part of our moral lives. The dominant agenda of bioethics—particularly in the current United States context—is of little use in guiding the relief of suffering, even though this task is at the heart of many of the issues that are brought to the court of bioethics. My goal is to show how the question of theodicy suggests a quite different agenda for bioethics.[1]

The Concept of Suffering

Although the relief of suffering has long been a goal of medicine, there have been relatively few efforts to explicate the concept of suffering in the medical and bioethical literature. This is likely due in part to the rather narrow way in which medicine primarily attends to suffering, namely, in relation to pathophysiological causes. It is also likely due to common perceptions of suffering as intensely personal and, therefore, highly variable. But some common features of suffering have been identified and they provide a conceptual basis for my discussion.[2]

Suffering is often distinguished from pain. There can be pain without suffering and vice versa. Pain, therefore, is neither a necessary nor a sufficient condition for suffering.[3] According to Eric Cassell, suffering occurs when, because of certain levels of pain or other circumstances, the "integrity or continued existence of the whole person" is threatened.[4] Suffering may arise when persons are unable to account for their causes of pain or the threats to their self-understanding,[5] the circumstances causing pain and suffering are beyond control,[6] persons' purposes are frustrated,[7] or persons are alienated from the relationships within which they are defined.[8]

What are thought to be common dimensions of suffering also point to the ways in which suffering is highly individual. "We do not suffer in general," as Stanley Hauerwas notes.[9] Exactly how an individual experiences suffering depends on how the sufferer interprets circumstances in relation to his or her self-understanding. These interpretations will be as unique as individuals are. This feature of suffering underlines the way in which suffering is said to alienate the self from others and even from the self. Others cannot fully share in the experience or understand its unique and complex features. Central to what the sufferer seeks by way of relief is a way of understanding that allows for a reintegration of self, a reconnection with others, and, if necessary, guidance in decisions regarding suffering.

What these dimensions of suffering point to, in short, is a search for meaning, and ultimately a search for goodness. As Erich Loewy has observed, "A critical component of suffering is its lack of meaning to the one suffering."[10] The term "meaning" is vague, but I shall refer to "meaning" as the intelligibility of suffering and the suffering self within a larger account of human goods and evils, such that goodness is not eliminated by suffering. Because of loss of control over the sources of suffering and threats to identity, relationships, and life goals, a sufferer is put in a position of searching for some way to make sense of what seems to be pointless and without purpose. Some sufferers may find that the convictions and narratives according to which they had previously understood the suffering and evils of humanity are unable to account for what afflicts them now. They face a personal kind of "epistemological crisis," to adapt Alasdair MacIntyre's term.[11] Those with less-developed means for interpreting suffering find themselves suffering further from a lack of epistemological resources to render their experience intelligible and meaningful. People literally suffer from lack of meaning and lack of relationships that can provide and affirm meaning—relationships with comforters as well as with communities of people whose lives bear witness to ways of accounting for the causes of suffering.

It is important at this point, however, to clarify that suffering is not eliminated through finding meaning alone. Relief of suffering is not reducible to an intellectual grasp of some account that lends meaning to it. I want to suggest, however, that *loss* of meaning is central to suffering, and that questions of theodicy and bioethics are related directly to that.

Medicine in Relation to Suffering

Modern Western medicine's central task has been to relieve suffering by eliminating physical maladies.[12] It has, in fact, developed a powerful array of technologies for this very purpose. A common criticism of medicine, however, is that it has become too narrowly focused on pathophysiology to the neglect of other components (e.g., psychological or environmental) of disease and suffering. To the extent this is true, medicine fails to address suffering even on medicine's own narrow terms.

In addition, medicine's tendency to address suffering too "biomedically" has led to another vein of criticism, namely, that medicine is increasingly guided by an imperative to apply itself indiscriminately to virtually all forms of human suffering. This motivation is captured by Gerald P. McKenny: "The imperative is to eliminate suffering and to expand the realm of human choice—in short, to relieve the human condition of subjection to the whims of fortune or the bonds of natural necessity."[13] Defending this thesis would require more space than I am able to give it and take me too far afield from my own argument. Many recent developments in medicine, however, lend validity to this critique: a growing range and use of psychopharmacological agents to "treat" undesirable behaviors or various forms of "unhappiness," manipulation of genetic material not just to treat but to "enhance" human capacities, physician involvement in suicide in the face of failures to provide adequate palliative care, prenatal genetic testing for a growing variety of conditions, discoveries of genetic processes by which aging occurs, and so on.

Medicine's current role in relieving suffering underlines its lack of internal standards and virtues and, therefore, of its own critical resources to address issues of meaning in suffering. Under the pressure of secular bioethics to respect patient autonomy, the primary goal of medicine has become to maximize individual choice with regard to well-being, with choice applied to a growing spate of human desires, in order to eliminate whatever a person, society, or medicine itself chooses to describe as suffering. Medicine, then, becomes a tradition by which all suffering is rendered pointless and subject to elimination—even to the extent of eliminating the sufferer. The current popular criticism of medicine as a primarily high-tech "curative" practice that is of little use to those suffering from chronic conditions largely confirms the critique of medicine's current imperative.

Medicine's primary role in relieving suffering, therefore, is to eliminate root physiological causes of suffering rather than to address the issues of meaning that suffering raises. According to some, this is as it should be, for medicine has no special expertise in addressing the search for meaning.[14] Such a tidy division is problematic, however. Biological and nonbiological dimensions of suffering are often intertwined in complex ways not easily perceived by the diagnostician. So-called psychological or spiritual forms of suffering often have physical manifestations that resist adequate treatment through biomedical means alone. Many of the patients—perhaps a majority—who sit before a physician suffer from maladies not reducible to biological components alone. And chronic conditions that resist cure cause forms of suffering that require a blend of technical medicine and a care that attends to personal matters of identity.

But, even if there is a defensible argument on behalf of a crude division of labor corresponding to a divided view of the self, there is another concern regarding medicine's current relation to suffering. Medicine's expanding charges to "relieve the human condition" and to maximize choice actually *reinforce* suffering because the first underlines suffering's essential pointlessness in all forms and the second, by leaving people to their choices, exacerbates suffering's tendency to isolate the sufferer from others. By failing to serve us in our efforts to relieve suffering by finding meaning in it, medicine subverts the ways in which illness and suffering are inscribed into the narratives and interpretive frameworks that can give them meaning.[15]

In fact, as medicine's imperative expands the ways in which we define disease and what is "normal" and "healthy," it increases the range of what we are told we suffer from.[16] The medicalization of many facets of human life—evidenced by such developments as the explosion of asserted genetic links not only to diseases but to virtually all traits and behaviors, the expansion of technical means of reproduction, the dominance of high-tech medicine at the end of life, and now the participation of medicine in suicide—entails that much more of our lives are subject to choices never before faced about medical control never before available. Increasingly, the suffering rooted in the "problems" of our finitude are created and defined by the medical diagnoses and "solutions" that are put before us. Ultimately, the underlying philosophy of medicine appears to be that there is nothing that human beings suffer from that is not, in principle, subject to elimination by medicine. Thus, medicine, by placing more of the conditions from which we ostensibly suffer into the realm of biology and thereby seeming to diminish human responsibility for these conditions, makes more of our suffering seem senseless because it apparently happens *to* us, rather than because of us.

It might be objected that this description of medicine in relation to suffering is too simple, that it is too distant from the ways in which health care professionals genuinely care for suffering patients in day-to-day clinical life. Certainly the contributions of medicine toward recognition and relief of suffering should not be discounted. Biomedical achievement as well as genuine compassion in medicine go a long way toward ameliorating suffering—the former in eliminating physiological causes and the latter in establishing a context of care and maintenance of some modicum of human relationship between the suffering person and the human community. Nevertheless, the growing dominance of the modern medical imperative entails that medicine is working at cross purposes in addressing suffering as one of its goals. To highlight this more starkly, I turn briefly to a reflection on a passage from literature.

Interlude: A Brief Commentary

Aldous Huxley's *Brave New World* is often invoked as a picture of how a society might look if advances in technology—particularly life science technology—were to succeed in offering us the best of what it portends, namely, elimination of virtually all undesirable contingencies of human biological finitude. Biotechnology enables social control to create a utopia: persons engineered for happiness, health, contentment with work, free and uncomplicated sexual relations, absence of ideological conflict, and death without discomfort or fear. On Huxley's planet, only certain designated areas called "reservations" are outside utopian engineering.

At one point in the story, a visitor, named "the Savage," from a reservation is visiting with Mustapha Mond, the "Controller" or supreme authority of the *Brave New World* civilization. The Savage is genuinely troubled and saddened by civilization's elimination of goods that come of the human struggle against the limiting conditions of human finitude.

> "You got rid of them. Yes, that's just like you. Getting rid of everything unpleasant instead of learning to put up with it. Whether 'tis better in the mind to suffer the slings and arrows of outrageous fortune, or to take arms against a sea of troubles and by opposing end them. . . . But you don't do either. Neither suffer nor oppose. You just abolish the slings and arrows. It's too easy."[17]

As the conversation continues, the sum of what the Savage is arguing for becomes poignantly clear.

> "Exposing what is mortal and unsure to all that fortune, death and danger dare, even for an egg-shell. Isn't there something in that?" he asked, looking up at Mustapha Mond. "Quite apart from God—though of course God would be a reason for it. Isn't there something in living dangerously?"
>
> "There's a great deal in it," the Controller replied. "Men and women must have their adrenals stimulated from time to time."
>
> "What?" questioned the Savage, uncomprehending.
>
> "It's one of the conditions of perfect health. That's why we've made the V.P.S. treatments compulsory."
>
> "V.P.S.?"
>
> "Violent Passion Surrogate. Regularly once a month. We flood the whole system with adrenin. It's the complete physiological equivalent of fear and rage. All the tonic effects of murdering Desdemona and being murdered by Othello, without any of the inconveniences."
>
> "But I like the inconveniences."
>
> "We don't," said the Controller. "We prefer to do things comfortably."
>
> "But I don't want comfort. I want God, I want poetry, I want real danger, I want freedom, I want goodness. I want sin."
>
> "In fact," said Mustapha Mond, "you're claiming the right to be unhappy."
>
> "All right then," said the Savage defiantly, "I'm claiming the right to be unhappy."
>
> "Not to mention the right to grow old and ugly and impotent; the right to have syphilis and cancer; the right to have too little to eat; the right to be lousy; the right to live in constant apprehension of what may happen to-morrow; the right to catch typhoid; the right to be tortured by unspeakable pains of every kind."
>
> There was a long silence.
>
> "I claim them all," said the Savage at last.
>
> Mustapha Mond shrugged his shoulders. "You're welcome," he said.[18]

Prior to this point in Huxley's story, the reader has likely been seduced by the attractiveness of the utopian society. The burdens of finitude are eliminated and human preferences are maximized. Nevertheless, it is difficult to resist a certain sympathy with the Savage's perspective. The reason for this sympathy lies in the ways in which we connect the goods and evils claimed by the Savage with our very humanity. The contingencies of human finitude that lead to sickness, conflict, and suffering of all kinds are also contingencies the struggle against which leads to or constitutes many of the goods we treasure—freedom, love, and justice, not to mention poetry, literature, and religion. Through such struggles and suffering we affirm our humanity, and the ways in which we resist contingencies define our moral character. My point is not to suggest the inherent goodness of suffering itself, but rather to affirm the conviction that to be human is to claim the contingencies of life, including and especially suffering, and to find meaning in the encounter with them. Our very capacities to experience suffering and enter into a caring relationship with those who suffer are central to our moral lives and human identity.[19]

Certainly the successes of medicine against disease and other causes of suffering exemplify the goods of struggle that the Savage's choice affirms. Yet, if we can also fairly say that medicine's pursuit of the elimination of suffering and the maximization of human choice is largely unlimited and unguided, then it not only tends in the direction of a *Brave New World* civilization as our future, but also conforms to and underwrites the ideology of such a civilization. Human identity and the goods we treasure are defined in part by the kinds of suffering we experience, our struggle against suffering, and how we situate it in contexts that provide meaning for it.

Huxley's utopia certainly depends on more than merely the availability of technologies that allow elimination of undesirable contingencies. However, the point of the story is not to depict historical inevitability but to critique efforts to deny our humanity. Huxley's utopia is, therefore, intended to be a negative one; it shows us what is at stake if we seek what medicine seems to be after. The appeal, however tiresome, to the lessons of *Brave New World* in the face of virtually every major advance of medicine and biotechnology cautions us to be mindful of this fact.

It is true that science and technology are unlikely ever to eliminate contingencies and conditions of finitude that lead to suffering. Theodicies of one sort or another will always be necessary. But, if our science and especially our medicine are to be guided ethically to places somewhere between utopian inhumanity and concession to true savagery, if they are to be defined by the meaning purchased through successful efforts against suffering rather than absolute denial of it, what will be the sources of such guidance?

The Limits of Bioethics

Gerald McKenny postulates two accounts of the origin of modern bioethics, the first a search for solutions to moral quandaries occasioned by modern technologies, and the second the need for a common morality to address a crisis in moral authority.[20] These two accounts are, of course, closely related. As technology in medicine and the life sciences posed new dilemmas, bioethics emerged to fill what appeared to be a vacuum in moral authority. That is, the resources of medicine were too thin to guide it into new territory, and the plurality of sources of moral authority in the larger society offered competing normative stances regarding how to advise medicine.

Through time, bioethics has evolved from an interdisciplinary conversation into a distinct discipline, accompanied now by increasing debate about matters of methodology, professional organization, and even certification. While its borders are still rough, its evolution testifies to certain dominant characteristics. The public discipline of bioethics in the United States relies on the tools of Anglo-American analytic philosophy to clarify concepts and create helpful distinctions, and on the use of "mid-level" moral principles to capture generic moral values that apply to medical practice. These devices are meant to obviate the need to appeal to more particularistic sources of moral authority and thus to have a wide appeal for a medical context increasingly characterized as interactions among strangers. This has also made bioethics appealing at the public policy level; its role, for example, in the National Institutes of Health's Human Embryo Research Panel and the National Bioethics Advisory Commission has further confirmed its kinship with the ethics and assumptions of American liberal polity and law.

Foremost among these assumptions is that respect for individual autonomy is the overriding value at stake in moral dilemmas. The elevation of autonomy to the status of a moral guide for medicine has done well in protecting individual patients from paternalism in the doctor-patient relationship and from restrictions on certain liberties that might be imposed by others with conflicting moral perspectives. But, as critics of present-day bioethics are beginning to point out, the ostensibly autonomous individual is left with little in the way of guidance, from either medicine or bioethics, about the development and use of medicine on the policy level and about treatment decisions on the individual level.

Even more significant, perhaps, is the way in which the so-called triumph of autonomy in bioethics has embodied a particular view of the self and personhood that is, after all, neither as neutral as claimed nor as benign as hoped. Gilbert Meilaender argues that, under bioethics' dominant methodology, "to be a person is to be, or have the capacity to be, an autonomous chooser, to take control over one's personal history, determining its bounds and limits."[21] In an autonomy-dominated ethics, moral decisions are made by the rational self in a moment of time, and the capacity for moral agency is the central feature of morality. The dominance of issues surrounding advance directives and informed consent highlights the degree to which a particular view of the person has taken hold in medical ethics. Absent, according to Meilaender, is any sense of the self as embodied, with a natural trajectory that extends over time.

The critical question for my argument then is, Do the assumptions of the dominant approach in bioethics have any contribution to make to questions about relief of the kind of suffering that raises issues of theodicy? Although not typically analyzed as such, the range of questions that engage bioethicists today largely have to do with the relief of suffering. These questions include not merely the typical spectrum of clinical quandaries—from treatment of extremely premature infants to adult end-of-life decision making—but also the guidance of personal as well as policy decisions regarding emerging medical technologies. Theodicy questions can arise for persons confronting decisions surrounding prenatal genetic testing, treatment options for infertility, fetal tissue transplantation for Parkinson's disease, and even technologies that promise to redefine current conditions of normality into conditions that we shall (in the future) suffer from. In all these situations one might ask, How can I account for what I suffer from, and what does my answer to that question suggest for what should I do about it? Can bioethics provide any answer to these questions, or any critical leverage to guide medicine in directions other than those required by its *Brave New World* imperative?

If we are to consider bioethics as a discipline that largely conforms to the assumptions and the resources of the liberal tradition—thereby maintaining a fictive neutrality with regard to views of personhood and individual autonomy—the answer to this last question must be no. Resolutions of most of the quandaries by which bioethics defines itself, however roughly, rely ultimately on assumptions that bioethics has mostly eschewed, such as normative conceptions of humanity and human relations, distinctive virtues and goals for medicine, social justice, and the necessity of reliance on rich traditions of morality. Yet such assumptions are at the heart of the following sorts of questions: How are we to regard the embryo, experimentation on which could lead to eradication of many causes of suffering? How are we to regard the genetically defective fetus, which is the source of much suffering for parents expecting their "perfect child"? How are we to consider technologies that may lead us to define our current aging process as something we should eliminate? How are we to care for the mentally handicapped person who is beyond the possibility of cure? And how are we to care for the terminally ill cancer patient whose life seems to him or her to be not worth living?

An autonomy-centered, public policy–oriented ethics is not likely have much to say about any of these problems. In fact, the autonomous individual is likely to find bioethics reinforcing the suffering found in these questions, insofar as autonomy, like suffering, essentially isolates the person from the relationships—intimate as well as communal—within which relief of suffering may be found.

Suffering is often seen as a threat to autonomy, rather than a source of it.[22] Yet, by finding meaning in suffering and making it part of our moral traditions, we develop mature resources to guide future judgments about resistance to suffering and its meaning.

Bioethics, far from providing critical leverage against the modern imperative of medicine, is more complicitous with it, for it "provides no moral framework within which to determine what kind of suffering should be eliminated and which choices are best."[23] This leaves medicine not only ethically liberated to eradicate whatever anyone considers a burden of finitude, but also positioned to define our preferences increasingly in the terms of an infinite progress that may ultimately redefine our humanity, if not deny it. At the same time, medicine neglects our responsibility to confront questions of meaning in ways that can inform our choices.[24]

Much more could be said about this than space allows. In fairness, many at work in the field of bioethics pursue agendas different from the one that has dominated the rise of a discipline so easily stereotyped. The remainder of my argument concerns how the question of theodicy may suggest and shape alternative approaches.

Theodicy as Relief of Suffering

Not all suffering will lead a person to raise the question of theodicy. How suffering is understood and experienced in individual cases determines whether theodicy becomes an issue. But if we can agree that suffering in certain contexts is constituted by a search for meaning, then theodicies represent a kind of relief of suffering.

The history of theodicy as a theological problem is long and complex; it also demonstrates the ways in which the form of this problem has been shaped by various ways of understanding God and rationality. So-called classic types of theodicy are attempts to put the burden of justifying individual instances of suffering in the context of the moral quality of a larger whole[25] and include such arguments as that evil is merely deprivation of good, or is instrumental for larger goods, or is only a partial vision of what is really good, and so on.[26]

In more recent discussions, the "problem of theodicy" has been seen as requiring a practical response, rather than a theoretical account. In this vein, medicine—or, more broadly, technology—has been called a theodicy of the modern era, enlisted by Western societies as their principal means of eliminating evil and suffering. I have argued above that such a view is problematic. Medicine is more like a "pretheodicy," removing causes of suffering in a way meant to preclude the encounter by the sufferer with the questions of meaning raised by suffering. As a kind of compassionate art, medicine at its best can play an important role in sufferers' quests for meaning by demonstrating care for them in ways that can facilitate their struggles to make sense of their suffering.

Some current writings on theodicy and suffering are critical of modern theodicies as attempts to rationalize what cannot be rationalized,[27] or even as sinful attempts to justify the ways of God to human beings. To construct a theodicy of the classical variety, the criticism goes, is to provide a universal answer for a problem that is necessarily individual and particular—individual as to the circumstances of suffering and particular as to the tradition of understanding in which God and/or the moral life is understood. There is no theodicy as such, because there is no suffering as such. As Hauerwas argues, to turn the theological problem of evil into a problem from anyone's perspective is to turn one's underlying faith into a system of beliefs knowable by anyone, and thereby to "underwrite the Enlightenment assumption that we are most fully ourselves when we are free of traditions and commitments other than those chosen from a position of complete autonomy."[28]

This line of criticism highlights the ways in which responses to suffering that enable the sufferer to find meaning in it depend on the connections that are made between the sufferer and traditions within which suffering and its relation to God and/or goodness are comprehended. Relief of suffering is found not in universality but through quite particular narratives of meaning and through relationships with persons in a context of care within which goodness is affirmed and narratives of meaning are realized concretely. The problem of theodicy in the experience of the sufferer is thus only partially an intellectual and abstract enterprise. Addressing it, however, may be a necessary step for avoiding despair.

For theologians and people of religious faith, the task is to seek new ways of intelligibly situating evolving medical realities of suffering within the narratives by which their faith communities are formed. They also must seek to build the communal relationships by which their convictions are lived out and sufferers are reminded of the traditions that grant their suffering meaning.

Bioethics lacks such resources. Yet the struggle with the question of theodicy does suggest areas for more concerted attention in bioethics if it is to have something to say about resistance to and relief of suffering.

The Challenge of Theodicy for Bioethics

It is clear that bioethics is not the sort of enterprise that can serve the sufferer by offering either a secular or a theological theodicy. A theodicy—a rich account of meaning for suffering—cannot be captured by a theory from nowhere. How can bioethics function as a public enterprise devoted to ethical guidance about issues of suffering without embracing a particular account of theodicy?

My analysis suggests a model for bioethics as a *mediator* of resources by which suffering can be informed and ultimately, one hopes, relieved. The resources for addressing the kinds of questions theodicies address point toward substantive insights that can guide both personal and policy judgments about the relief of suffering, as well as about how to live with the sorts of suffering that are inevitable in human life. This mediating endeavor implies a different kind of agenda for bioethics than that which currently defines its dominant approach, one that would consist as much in identifying appropriate questions to ask as in providing normative recommendations. What are the elements of an agenda that could fulfill this mediating role?

1. The first major component suggested by theodicies is essentially anthropological, namely, an effort to provide some initial step in accounting for suffering by considering how it is constitutive of human life. This would entail not merely more rigorous analysis of the concept of suffering as such but, more important, exploration of how suffering is understood in relation to various conceptions of human nature. The questions to ask are: What is suffering? What are its sources and its forms? What are its roles within ways of living a human life? How does it participate in defining us as human?

2. Theodicies also challenge us to confront the ethical task of situating suffering in relation to goodness and our moral perspectives and ways of life, that is, of exploring the relations between suffering and our moral traditions so that suffering can be seen to be compatible with goodness and relevant to how we construe our lives morally. This work involves drawing connections between the rich theological and philosophical accounts of suffering in human existence and the ethical terrain that defines bioethics. The normative implications of these accounts can inform judgments about how suffering can be meaningfully accepted or how it should be resisted, and with what ethical guidance or constraints.

3. In a general way, bioethics can bring these resources to bear critically on the modern imperative of medicine and on the ways in which medicine and the social values that drive it may, in some respects, reinforce suffering rather than accommodate judgments about kinds of suffering and their meaning. Bioethics should press questions about the sort of tradition medicine is and is becoming, questions related to its context of care in encounter with suffering persons. As McKenny has shown,[29] a variety of theoretical approaches, elaborated by particular thinkers, are available as resources for such a critique: those that consider the normative conception of the human (e.g., Hans Jonas and James Gustafson), the telos of medicine itself and the goods of its practice (e.g., Leon Kass and Stanley Hauerwas), appeals to norms of the common good (e.g., Daniel

Callahan), phenomenologies of the body (e.g., Drew Leder and Richard Zaner), and the moral significance of the body (e.g., Gerald McKenny).

4. Of course, social practices such as medicine are also formed and reformed continually by the social values that constitute its larger context. Part of the critique of medicine, then, must involve criticism of the ways in which the values of society create and reinforce the suffering encountered in medicine and the ways in which medicine and life-science technology respond to them. Central to this effort are considerations of how human evil, and not God, is responsible for much of the suffering that we now consider to be merely material or biological. Social values surrounding human health, beauty, and well-being are implicated in our modern conceptions of suffering, as is a faith in progress informed largely by technological development.[30]

5. A more specific anthropological task for bioethics, suggested by theodicies in regard to medical suffering, would be further exploration of the meanings of embodiment. This would involve an effort to "become aware of the attitudes and practices that have formed us in connection with the technological control of medicine over our bodies and to determine which attitudes and practices should form us."[31] Such an effort could provide a critique of evolving "normalizing" standards that medicine and social values impose on us, and point us to alternative traditions of interpretation. It would bring into question assumptions—especially within the dominant approach of bioethics itself—about the relation of embodiment to personhood that currently plague many bioethical debates.

6. Finally, not merely matters of justice but also dimensions of care are suggested by theodicy. Theodicy especially points bioethical considerations of care in the direction of the chronically ill, insofar as chronic conditions are forms of tragedy that evoke questions of theodicy as well as of ongoing care. Much of the goodness sought in relief of suffering comes through the binding of the suffering person in relationships both with those offering care in the immediate circumstances and with broader communities. Attention on both clinical and policy levels to the dynamics of such relationships and how they might be supported would be an integral part of a revised agenda for bioethics.

Methodological Note

A couple of methodological implications of my analysis should also be made explicit. The highly variable ways in which suffering is understood in individual cases, as well as the narrative character of many traditions that lend meaning to suffering, entail that bioethics will have to attend to narrative. The ways in which suffering is comprehended are often captured in narrative traditions, like religions. In addition, people make sense of their own suffering by seeking to understand it within the story and stories of their own lives, relying on both past perspectives and future hopes. Exploration of how suffering is understood will often have to rely on techniques of narrative analysis.

Moreover, the types of explorations required to address suffering are best served by interdisciplinary analysis, rather than from within the conceptual and methodological parameters of a single discipline. A bioethics constructed as an intersection not merely of distinct disciplines, but also of distinct traditions of thought, would be more adequate to the descriptive and normative tasks implicated in the search for relief of suffering.

Conclusion

Persons will not always be able to find meaning in their suffering, but the attempt to do so creates challenges for our thinking about efforts to overcome suffering. I have argued that the kind of problem theodicy represents sets us to tasks that press our bioethical thinking to explore the geographies of suffering. Theodicy points us in the direction of resources that enable persons to find meaning in their suffering and that provide critical leverage against medicine's imperative to deny any meaning or humanity in suffering at all.

It is perhaps ultimately through the relationships that suffering people can maintain with others that their suffering will be most adequately addressed. Bioethics will be of small use in that. But to the extent that bioethics can address the reasons why people suffer and how that suffering can possibly be compatible with the goodness we seek in life, it will offer real guidance in the choices people and societies make to relieve suffering.

Conclusion:
Pain Seeking Understanding

Margaret E. Mohrmann

The chapters in this book identify various voices of pain and suffering, especially those associated with more or other than physical misery. They show both that the voices are speaking to medicine, whether medicine wishes to hear them or not, and that there is a significant spiritual component to suffering for many, perhaps most, people. These chapters also consider ways of construing suffering that may prove illuminating for those who suffer and those who seek to help them. From logical arguments to practical suggestions, from theological anthropology to chaos theory, from syllogisms to stories and art, the various modes of grasping and working through difficult central questions arising from the fact of pain here form a whole that gives shape and substance to theodicy as it is experienced and enacted in daily life.

The book, having stressed the significance of both the questions and the responses involved in thinking about or "doing" theodicy, creates puzzles of its own. How can those who tend to the ill and injured be selected, or taught, or encouraged to be responsible clinicians, able to respond to the depth of their patients' suffering, able to be responsive to the vital and sometimes frightening puzzles exposed by pain seeking understanding. This epilogue specifically considers these challenges to medical education and biomedical ethics.

As the preceding chapters emphasize, common factors in the queries of those who suffer include the elements of tragedy: the inescapable fact of the suffering, the haunting awareness of choices made and demanded, the confusion of being enmeshed in a situation that surpasses comprehension. Common aspects of the kind of responsiveness suggested for clinicians are expressed in recurring words and phrases: hearing, receiving, holding patient stories; respectful witnessing; being fully present, open both to disturbing inquiries and to the possibility of mediating consolation; accepting expressions of non-sense, honoring them as paradoxically meaningful; offering oneself, or someone else, as companion for the quest.

The vocation of medicine may be a "solution" of sorts to the secular problem of evil, as asserted here by Nelson. It may also be a significant part of a response to the religious problem of evil, insofar as practitioners, along with their patients, can attentively and faithfully hold together, as Bouchard suggests and others echo, fragments of belief and experience, none of which is less real for being apparently irreconcilable with the others. But, how does one find or form clinicians who can and will be so receptive, so ready not only to tolerate but to validate paradox?

There are at least three phases, broadly defined, in determining the character, attitudes, and approaches of physicians: selection, education, and experience. Controversy has long existed, and surely will persist, about which stage is critical for development of the sort of doctor that suffering seems to need.

The process of selection for medical school engenders its own particular set of questions. Many argue that because most students, in the United States at least, enter medical school in their twenties, their moral formation is virtually complete; their personalities and attitudes are superficially modifiable but basically fixed. Just as a theodicy that insists upon preserving God's sovereignty or one that focuses instead on God's participation in pain may reflect as much about the psychology and experiences of the theologian arguing the case as about the nature of God, so a doctor's ability or inability to attend well to suffering may have more to do with his or her own personality traits and background, including religious formation, than with anything gleaned from medical education, ethics, or patient encounters.

If this is the case, should medical school admission committees then be screening applicants for traits and prior experiences or education that may be thought to characterize physicians able to respond to suffering? Who decides what those traits and teachings are? (A related question is whether such committees should be composed entirely of medical professionals selecting their students and future colleagues, or should include laypersons selecting their future physicians.) How can the desired characteristics be accurately identified? Some medical school applicants are adept at discovering and then claiming personal attributes sought by the schools to which they apply. What, then, would it mean to look for "true" responsibility? Should the gatekeepers of medical schools rely on personality inventories or hone their interviewing skills? What questions would one ask? Even if it were thought possible to define clearly the desired traits and to screen accurately for them, *should* that be done? Does medicine thereby risk losing a critical level of diversity among its practitioners? That is, would such a selection process weed out some future researchers or physicians who do not see patients but who carry out tasks, such as pathological studies, necessary for the practice of good clinical medicine by others?

On the other hand, it has long been recognized that students entering medical school, no matter their age or personalities, have little notion of what it is to practice medicine, and that most are open to learning what doctors do and how they do it. Thus, many would argue that medical education and the apprenticeship period of residency training are crucial for determining students' ability to perceive and accept the sorts of professional roles outlined in this book, even if that ability is configured to some extent by vagaries of personality and culture. If this is the case, the question becomes whether and how one can teach a student doctor to be a respectful witness. Such a curriculum might require each instructor, of biochemistry as well as pediatrics, to be aware of what she or he is teaching about doctoring while imparting facts about amino acids or inborn metabolic disease.

If clinical responsibility to suffering is to be taught by medical school faculty, how are the teachers to be selected and/or trained? Even a superficial survey of academic physicians would identify many who are themselves apparently unprepared to recognize or accept spiritual queries from their patients. Is it enough that students be exposed to an occasional doctor who does manifest the openness to incomprehensible pain and indeterminate causation that human suffering requires of its witnesses? How many such exposures are necessary for effective teaching, especially when placed over against the examples of other faculty members who deny any role for the clinician in attending to suffering that is not clearly physical?

Many doctors who serve as respectful witnesses of their patients' pain readily admit that they were taught to do so by the patients themselves. That is, it may be clinical experience that is the best and perhaps the only effective teacher of responsibility. However, just as chance favors the prepared mind, so clinical experience can teach only the receptive mind. Should medical educators, at a minimum, be reminding students that thoughtful and compassionate responsiveness to suffering is an integral part of good medical practice and that they must be willing to let patients show them what that entails? Perhaps each instructor could be charged with telling students, as often as seems necessary, that the academic focus on facts and answers, data and outcomes, can rarely speak intelligibly to the phenomena of suffering. Such cautions, like a memento mori, might counterbalance the prevailing emphasis in medicine on total comprehension and control with a category of virtually universal human experience that, by definition, resists understanding. Perhaps this could free the doctor-in-training to focus on the patient's experience and dilemma rather than on the clinician's own need to provide answers or remedies.

David Morris, as part of his argument for the heuristic value of tragedy in the approach to medical suffering, claims:

> What we learn from tragedy . . . does not always resemble a nugget of portable wisdom ("the moral of the story"). It is sometimes more like an experience that changes you in ways you cannot exactly explain.[1]

Clinical experience can be transformative. It is not just that good clinicians can learn from each patient some "pearl" (medical jargon for "a nugget of portable wisdom") to inform and enhance future practice. A responsible clinician also recognizes that one courts profound personal change by standing still in the midst of tragedy, with open eyes and heart, allowing oneself to be moved. A good clinical teacher helps students recognize and address their fear, often disguised as intellectual disdain or as professional concern for maintaining boundaries, of vulnerability to such a change, by teaching and demonstrating that the transformation, far from being destructive, enriches the skills and the person of the physician. Facing the realities of tragedy—unfairness, accountability, intolerable randomness, the exposure of previously untested and now unsustainable beliefs about God and the cosmos—is the route to a richer comprehension of one's own life and beliefs, and of one's vocation.

Whether such a transformation by clinical experience can occur often depends on the clinician's being prepared and willing to face the darkness at the edge, at the boundary not between patient and doctor but between known and unknown. The physician, or nurse, or chaplain must acknowledge that the abyss is not her or his own now, although some day it may be, and then must be brave enough to accompany the patient along that edge with attentive presence and care.

> To use Tillich's phrase, the physician works *on the boundary* between the promise of human creativity and the ultimate lack of sovereignty characteristic of human finitude. Correspondingly, the role of the physician is not only to rally patients in their struggles, but also to assist them through the inevitable transitions of life, including the passage into death. Physicians no less than ministers are challenged to have zest and talent for both roles, and to be able to change roles when struggle must give way to acquiescence, embrace to relinquishment.[2]

In this book, Anderson recalls for us the distinction, drawn in Reinhold Niebuhr's "Serenity Prayer," between those things that befall us that call for courage to resist and change, and those things that, because they cannot be changed, require that the struggle "give way to acquiescence." When I speak of transformation occurring at the still point in the middle of tragic events, I do not imply that the tragedy itself, the suffering can necessarily be altered. Rather, it is the person suffering and the person witnessing who can be changed. Niebuhr explains, by means of his prayer, that wisdom is required to distinguish between experiences that need brave resistance and those that need calm acceptance. The transformation that tragedy can work in us is a growth in wisdom.

It seems to me that precisely here is where one can speak of the role of medical ethics, and the implications for the discipline that arise from the discussions collected in this book. For who within the profession of medicine, if not ethics, can be the voice of tragedy and uncertainty, of the obligation to be brave and present in the face of those trials, of the possibility and goodness of being transformed by clinical experience?

Richard Selzer eloquently argues that one learns compassion—the ability and inclination to share the experience of suffering with one's patient in substantive ways—only gradually and cumulatively through practicing medicine:

> No easy shaft of grace this. . . . Slowly it gathers . . . until, at last, it is a pure call-
> ing . . . telling that out of the resonance between the sick man and the one who
> tends him there may spring that profound courtesy that the religious call Love.[3]

This kind of language—words of courtesy and love—is not often heard in the lecture halls of academic medicine. It is the language spoken by religion, by literature, and by ethics. If we in medicine are to hear and recognize the call Selzer is referring to, the call that arises from encounters with our patients, then our ears must be schooled by religion, or the humanities, or ethics, for science cannot teach us this truth.

Within most medical schools religion can have little to say, given our secular and pluralist culture; a religious tradition may speak clearly to its followers, among them clinicians, but often has few opportunities to speak immediately to doctors attending to the sorts of medical tragedies with which we are here concerned. The humanities may and certainly should have some voice in medical education, but the extent to which that voice is heard and honored is variable at best. The only nonscientific voice given serious attention within medicine currently is biomedical ethics, which is, therefore, obligated to act as a mediator of the sort Mark Hanson describes in his chapter: a mediator of rich traditions of spiritual and moral thought—religions, philosophies, and the literature of tragedy—which can speak to physicians and their patients at the boundaries of human comprehension and endurance.

In this sense, ethics can serve as the "conscience" of medical education and medical practice, reminding us continually of the professional and personal moral obligation to stay with our patients in their boundary experiences. Ethics must call us back again and again to our primary obligation to the patient before us, not to our own needs, however urgent, to escape the evidence of non-sense invading reality, the appalling consequences of apparently trivial choices, the distressing struggles of pain seeking understanding.

It is ethics that must help clinicians learn how to work through our own spiritual dilemmas in the face of suffering so that we may be able to hear those of our patients without being compelled to impose the quieting constructions we have devised for ourselves. Even when *my* beliefs insist that no God worthy of the name would inflict a painful and crippling disease on a child—or on anyone else, for that matter—in order to work out some divine plan of complex good, I cannot turn away from or attempt to derail that child's parents' attempts to understand the catastrophe as being somehow within God's will. Ethics reminds me that part of my task as their child's doctor is to accompany them in their struggles, not to engage them in mine.

It is not that bioethics should no longer be concerned with policy making, or the encroachments of capitalism on an enterprise that cannot be commodified without fundamental distortion, or the sorts of end-of-life dilemmas that preoccupy many ethics committees. Rather, ethics in medicine must *also* recognize its role in mediating to this self-consciously scientific discipline the rich understandings of self, human life, and the divine that can support and teach—even transform—individual clinicians as we face the daily encounter with evil suffered by human bodies and minds. These are the understandings that also nurture the patients for whom we care; the common ground patient and clinician can find within various ways of ordering the cosmos may help us together hold the paradoxical fragments of a life broken apart by senseless and incomprehensible pain. That holding together is an enactment of the "profound courtesy" of which Selzer speaks. Courtesy is the very core of human ethics, and ethics should tell us constantly that profound courtesy, which "the religious call Love," is also the very core of the practice of moral medicine.

Notes

Introduction: Suffering, Medicine, and Faith

1. *The Oxford Dictionary of the Christian Church*, 2d ed., ed. F. L. Cross and E. A. Livingstone (Oxford: Oxford University Press, 1974), s.v. "theodicy."

2. Tyron L. Inbody, in *The Transforming God: An Interpretation of Suffering and Evil* (Louisville: Westminster John Knox Press, 1997), 30, distinguishes the traditional logical problem of reconciling evil with divine omnipotence and goodness from a broader sense of theodicy as "the effort to *understand* the occurrence and place of evil within one's larger theological framework which defines and describes what one believes about God and the world."

3. See, in this book, Elliot Dorff's chapter, "Rabbi, Why Does God Make Me Suffer?" and Harold S. Kushner, *When Bad Things Happen to Good People* (New York: Avon, 1983).

4. Particularly helpful discussions of various ways of "solving" the enigma of theodicy, in which the balance struck among divine goodness, omnipotence, and earthly evil by each theory is clearly drawn, are found in *Encountering Evil: Live Options in Theodicy*, ed. Stephen T. Davis (Atlanta: John Knox Press, 1981). An excellent brief review and critique is David H. Smith's chapter, "Suffering, Medicine, and Christian Theology," in *On Moral Medicine: Theological Perspectives in Medical Ethics*, ed. Stephen E. Lammers and Allen Verhey (Grand Rapids, Mich.: Eerdmans, 1987), 255–61.

5. For discussions of the free-will defense, see Stephen T. Davis, "Free Will and Evil," in *Encountering Evil*, 69–99, and C. S. Lewis's classic apology, *The Problem of Pain* (New York: Macmillan, 1962).

6. John H. Hick is perhaps the best-known proponent of this view. See his "An Irenaean Theodicy," in *Encountering Evil*, 39–68, as well as his longer work, *Evil and the God of Love* (New York: Harper & Row, 1978).

7. Smith, "Suffering, Medicine, and Christian Theology," 257.

8. C. S. Lewis, in *The Great Divorce* (New York: Macmillan, 1963), 67, makes this point clear: "Both good and evil, when they are full grown, become retrospective.... All this earthly past will have been Heaven to those who are saved. ... That is what mortals misunderstand. They say of some temporal suffering, 'No future bliss can make up for it,' not knowing that Heaven, once attained, will work backwards and turn even that agony into a glory."

9. See John K. Roth, "A Theodicy of Protest," in *Encountering Evil*, 7–37, and the novels of Elie Wiesel.

10. Among numerous examples of this sort of theodicy, see Wendy Farley, *Tragic Vision and Divine Compassion: A Contemporary Theodicy* (Louisville: Westminster/John Knox

Press, 1990); Tyron L. Inbody, *The Transforming God*; and David R. Griffen, "Creation out of Chaos and the Problem of Evil," in *Encountering Evil*, 101–36.

11. John B. Cobb Jr., "The Problem of Evil and the Task of Ministry," in *Encountering Evil*, 167.

1. Holding Fragments

1. See Kenneth Surin, *Theology and the Problem of Evil* (Oxford: Basil Blackwell, 1986), especially ch. 4; Wendy Farley, *Tragic Vision and Divine Compassion: A Contemporary Theodicy* (Louisville: Westminster/John Knox Press, 1990); Paul Ricoeur, "Evil, a Challenge to Philosophy and Theology," *Journal of the American Academy of Religion* 53 (1985): 635–50. See also Mark I. Wallace, *Fragments of the Spirit: Nature, Violence, and the Renewal of Creation* (New York: Continuum, 1996), 189 ff., where he describes Paul Ricoeur's recent writings on evil and wisdom literature as "theodicy in a practical register."

2. On juxtaposing "fragments," see Emil Fackenheim, *God's Presence in History: Jewish Affirmations and Philosophical Reflections* (New York: Harper & Row, 1970). While I do not limit the fragments to scripture and commentary, some may find such juxtaposing to be "midrashic"; Esther Menn called my attention to Daniel Boyarin, "Voices in the Text: Midrash and the Inner Tension of Biblical Narrative," *Revue biblique* 93–94 (1986): 581–97. On suffering being incommensurate with theory, see Theodor Adorno, *Negative Dialectics*, trans. E. B. Ashton (New York: Continuum, 1983).

3. Jesus' own rhetorical implication is not immediately clear. The entire passage reads (RSV), "'Doubtless you will quote to me this proverb, "Physician heal yourself; what we have heard you did at Capernaum, do here also in your own country."' And he said, 'Truly, I say to you, no prophet is acceptable in his own country.'" Implicitly, the people long for healing yet resent and disbelieve.

4. See Elaine Scarry, *The Body in Pain: The Making and Unmaking of the World* (New York: Oxford University Press, 1985), especially the introduction.

5. Margaret E. Mohrmann, *Medicine as Ministry: Reflections on Suffering, Ethics, and Hope* (Cleveland: The Pilgrim Press, 1995), 115.

6. See Larry D. Bouchard, *Tragic Method and Tragic Theology: Evil in Contemporary Drama and Religious Thought* (University Park: Pennsylvania State University Press, 1989), especially ch. 1; and my entry, "Tragedy," in the *Encyclopedia of Bioethics*, rev. ed. (New York: Macmillan, 1995), 5: 2490–96.

7. Paul Ricoeur, *The Symbolism of Evil*, trans. Emerson Buchanan (Boston: Beacon, 1967), 212.

8. Martha C. Nussbaum, *The Fragility of Goodness: Luck and Ethics in Greek Tragedy and Philosophy* (Cambridge: Cambridge University Press, 1986), esp. 122–35.

9. See Wendy Doniger O'Flaherty, *The Origins of Evil in Hindu Mythology* (Berkeley: University of California Press, 1976).

10. For a discussion of Hebrew laments, which occur in the prophets, Lamentations, and Job as well as in Psalms, see Bernhard W. Anderson, *Out of the Depths: The Psalms Speak for Us Today*, rev. ed. (Philadelphia: Westminster Press, 1983), ch. 3. See also Dietrich

Bonhoeffer, *Prayerbook of the Bible: An Introduction to the Psalms*, trans. James H. Burtness, in *Dietrich Bonhoeffer Works*, vol. 5 (Minneapolis: Fortress Press, 1996), 169.

11. For contrasting views of anxiety, sin, and tragic contingency, see Reinhold Niebuhr, *The Nature and Destiny of Man*, vol. 1 (New York: Scribners, 1941), esp. 180–85; and Edward Farley, *Good and Evil* (Minneapolis: Fortress Press, 1990), ch. 6. Both trace their interpretations to Soren Kierkegaard's *The Concept of Anxiety*, ed. and trans. Reidar Thomte and Albert B. Anderson (Princeton, N.J.: Princeton University Press, 1980).

12. See Fackenheim, *God's Presence in History*, 69; and what the Rebbe says in Elie Wiesel's novel *The Gates of the Forest* (New York: Schocken, 1964), 198.

13. I owe this use of "rupture" to Susan E. Shapiro, in "Hearing the Testimony of Radical Negation," *Concilium* 175 (1984): 3–10. On "irretrievable loss," I am grateful to Jonathan Sherwood's dissertation in progress on Paul Celan.

14. William C. Placher, *The Domestication of Transcendence: How Modern Thinking about God Went Wrong* (Louisville: Westminster John Knox Press, 1996).

15. See Surin, *Theology and the Problem of Evil*, 42–52.

16. See, for example, Langdon Gilkey, *Message and Existence: An Introduction to Christian Theology* (New York: Seabury, 1979); Johan Baptist Metz, *Faith in History and Society: Toward a Practical Fundamental Theology*, trans. David Smith (New York: Seabury, 1980); Edward Farley, *Divine Empathy* (Minneapolis: Fortress Press, 1996).

17. See Bouchard, *Tragic Method*, 226–27.

18. William Nicholson, *Shadowlands: A Play* (London: Samuel French, 1990). My comments, while referring to Lewis's writing, are directed only to the play and its characters. I am not concerned here, as others will surely be, with whether any version of *Shadowlands* is true to the biographies and temperaments of Lewis and Davidman.

19. Nicholson, *Shadowlands*, 2. This argument, that suffering effects "soul-making," closely follows C. S. Lewis, *The Problem of Pain* (1940; New York: Macmillan, 1962), especially ch. 6.

20. Nicholson, *Shadowlands*, 30. See C. S. Lewis, *A Grief Observed* (1961; New York: Bantam, 1976), 31–32.

21. Nicholson, *Shadowlands*, 47.

22. God is no longer the "Cosmic Sadist" but the "great iconoclast," who shatters human images of moral goodness (*Grief Observed*, 76). For criticism of *A Grief Observed*, see John Beversluis, *C. S. Lewis and the Search for Rational Religion* (Grand Rapids, Mich.: Eerdmans, 1985), 150–61; on *The Problem of Pain*, see Austin Farrer, "The Christian Apologist," in *Light on C. S. Lewis*, ed. Jocelyn Gibb (London: Geoffrey Bles, 1965), 31–43.

23. Nicholson, *Shadowlands*, 53. See Lewis, *Grief Observed*, 52, 85–86.

24. On being a messenger to God, see Wiesel, *Gates of the Forest*, 225–26. Wiesel reports the trial in his narrative *Night*, and he resituates it in the play *The Trial of God*. When interviewed in the *Long Search* film series (*The Chosen People*, 1978), Wiesel said that after the trial the participants prayed.

25. Quotations are from Tony Kushner, "A Prayer," in *Thinking about the Longstanding Problems of Virtue and Happiness: Essays, a Play, Two Poems, and a Prayer* (New York: Theatre Communications Group, 1995), 217–24.

26. See John Levenson, *Creation and the Persistence of Evil: The Jewish Drama of Divine Omnipotence* (San Francisco: Harper & Row, 1988), esp. ch. 2–4.

27. This discussion refers to Matthew, ch. 27; Mark, ch. 15; and Luke 22:66–23:48.

28. Jürgen Moltmann, *The Crucified God*, trans. R. A. Wilson and John Bowden (New York: Harper & Row, 1973), 252.

29. Fackenheim, *God's Presence in History*, 77.

30. I am grateful to James Duke, Margaret Galloway, Jennifer Geddes, Charles Mathewes, Margaret Mohrmann, Peter Ochs, Eugene Rogers, and members of the Association of Disciples for Theological Discussion, who were gracious enough to read and offer critical comments on this work.

3. The Tragedy of "Why Me, Doctor?"

1. Larry D. Bouchard, "Tragedy," in *Encyclopedia of Bioethics*, rev. ed. (New York: Macmillan, 1995), 5: 2490–96.

2. Harmon L. Smith and Larry R. Churchill, *Professional Ethics and Primary Care Medicine* (Durham, N.C.: Duke University Press, 1986).

3. Reynolds Price, *A Whole New Life* (New York: Atheneum, 1994), 53.

4. Rita Charon, Joanne T. Banks, Julia E. Connelly, et al., "Literature and Medicine: Contributions to Clinical Practice," *Annals of Internal Medicine* 122 (1995): 599–606.

5. Gregory S. Orr, *A Preface to Poetry* (Charlottesville: University of Virginia Printing and Copying Services, 1997), 1–38.

6. Julia E. Connelly, "The Whole Story: Tolstoy's *The Death of Ivan Ilyich* and Olsen's 'Tell Me a Riddle,'" *Literature and Medicine* 9 (1990): 150–61.

4. When Truth Is Mediated by a Life

1. Donald P. Spence, *Narrative Truth and Historical Truth: Meaning and Interpretation in Psychoanalysis* (New York: Norton, 1982).

2. Alasdair MacIntyre, *After Virtue*, 2d ed. (Notre Dame, Ind.: University of Notre Dame Press, 1984), 187 ff.

3. *Chaos and Complexity: Scientific Perspectives on Divine Action*, ed. Robert John Russell, Nancey Murphy, and Arthur R. Peacocke (Vatican City State: Vatican Observatory; Berkeley, Calif.: Center for Theology and the Natural Sciences, 1995).

4. James M. Gustafson, *Ethics from a Theocentric Perspective*, 2 vols. (Chicago: University of Chicago Press, 1981 and 1984).

5. William F. May, *The Patient's Ordeal* (Bloomington: Indiana University Press, 1991), 14.

6. Paul Ricoeur, *Time and Narrative*, vol. 1 (Chicago: University of Chicago Press, 1984), 65.

5. Someone Is Always Playing Job

1. Archibald MacLeish, *J.B.* (Boston: Houghton Mifflin, 1986), 11.

2. Deborah E. Healey, "Painful Stories, Moments of Grace"; Julia E. Connelly, "The Tragedy of 'Why Me, Doctor?'"; Albert H. Keller, "When Truth Is Mediated by a Life."

3. See, for example, several chapters in *Encountering Evil: Live Options in Theodicy*, ed. Stephen T. Davis (Atlanta: John Knox Press, 1981), and, in this book, the chapter by Daniel Sulmasy, "Finitude, Freedom, and Suffering."

4. David Morris, *The Culture of Pain* (Berkeley: University of California Press, 1991), 18. Several pages later he makes a comment directly relevant to the case just presented: "I would propose that while the doctor typically approaches pain as a puzzle or challenge, the patient typically experiences it as a mystery"(25).

5. Adrienne Rich has said that "until we can understand the assumptions in which we are drenched, we cannot know ourselves" (*On Lies, Secrets, and Silence: Selected Prose 1966–1978* [New York: Norton, 1979], 35). The assumptions about God that comprise our interpretive matrix are built up over time, not only from church teachings and liturgy, but also and especially by our experiences of good and evil, of love and distance, of relation and isolation. Inevitably, one's personality traits also significantly color the tendency to form certain assumptions and not others—e.g., the readiness to see love at work in suffering or to interpret pain as deserved punishment.

6. Leo Tolstoy, *The Death of Ivan Ilych*, trans. Lynn Solotaroff (New York: Bantam, 1981), 66, 89, 96–97.

7. Despite the intellectual inadequacy of Alvin Plantinga's explanation that the evil of physical suffering is due to the malign actions of fallen angels (in *God, Freedom, and Evil* [Grand Rapids, Mich.: Eerdmans, 1974]; see Sulmasy, "Finitude"), Connelly's example reveals the proximity of Plantinga's claim to some popular theology.

8. Sebastian Faulks, *Birdsong* (London: Vintage, 1994), 232. In a similar vein, Madame Blavatsky, the nineteenth-century doyenne of theosophy, once said: "I used to wonder at and pity the people who sell their souls to the Devil, but now I only pity them. They do it to have somebody on their side" (cited in Seamus Heaney, "All Ireland's Band," *Atlantic Monthly* 280 [November 1997]: 156).

9. As J.B. cries, "What I *can't* bear is the blindness—meaninglessness—the numb blow fallen in the stumbling night" (MacLeish, *J.B.*, 108).

10. Tyron L. Inbody, *The Transforming God: An Interpretation of Suffering and Evil* (Louisville: Westminster John Knox Press, 1997), 116: "The problem at the center of much of the lament tradition [bemoaning the "shadow side of God"] may not be so much the character of God as it is the 'cognitive dissonance' between what we experience of God in the real world and what we are taught by our religious and theological tradition we are to believe."

11. MacLeish, *J.B.*, 12.

12. Martha Nussbaum, *Love's Knowledge: Essays on Philosophy and Literature* (New York: Oxford University Press, 1990), 5–7 and throughout.

13. Richard Selzer, *Mortal Lessons: Notes on the Art of Surgery* (New York: Simon & Schuster, 1976), 46.

14. Larry D. Bouchard, "Tragedy," in *Encyclopedia of Bioethics*, rev. ed. (New York: Macmillan, 1995), 5: 2490–96. See also his thoughtful and provocative work *Tragic Method and Tragic Theology: Evil in Contemporary Drama and Religious Thought* (University Park: Pennsylvania State University Press, 1989).

15. Morris, *Culture of Pain*, 244–45. On page 245, citing others on the subject of why medicine ignores suffering, Morris concludes that, "Suffering in effect proves too hard to measure." It would be a salutary outcome indeed if the patent truth of that statement were to stop physicians from trying to force patients' experiences of pain onto a digital grid (i.e., "On a scale of one to ten, how bad is your pain?"), a vacuous exercise that cannot be answered accurately by anyone, cannot provide a meaningful understanding of pain and its associated suffering, and must serve only to relieve the physician's impatient anxiety in the face of something inherently nonquantifiable and closed to modern techniques of chemical analysis or imaging.

16. Bouchard, "Tragedy," 2494.

17. Wendy Farley, "Beyond Sociology: Studies of Tragedy, Sin, and Symbols of Evil," review of (among others) *Escape from Paradise: Evil and Tragedy in Feminist Theology*, by Kathleen M. Sands, in *Religious Studies Review* 22 (1996): 126.

18. See, for example, Eric Cassell, "The Nature of Suffering and the Goals of Medicine," *New England Journal of Medicine* 306 (1982): 639–45.

19. In an interesting and illuminating return to a Dickensian novelistic ethos, such works as Dorothy Allison's *Bastard out of Carolina* (New York: Dutton, 1992) and Jane Hamilton's *The Book of Ruth* (Boston: Houghton, Mifflin, 1988) detail the hardscrabble lives of persons not generally encountered in mainstream literature.

20. Douglas John Hall, *God and Human Suffering: An Exercise in the Theology of the Cross* (Minneapolis: Augsburg, 1986), 90.

21. George Macdonald, from *David Elginbrod*, bk. 1, chapter 13, as cited in *Bartlett's Familiar Quotations*, 15th ed., ed. E. M. Beck (Boston: Little, Brown, 1980), 594–95.

22. Hall, for example, in *God and Human Suffering* cites the ancient Jewish understanding that God's distance from creation is ethical, but not physical (112). Jesus' cry from the cross, lamenting and questioning God's absence from his pain, seals the Christian conviction that God has received into God's self—and there remembers—the profound loneliness and wracking, wordless pain that comprise human suffering.

23. Morris, *Culture of Pain*, 253, 255.

24. H. Richard Niebuhr, *The Responsible Self* (New York: Harper & Row, 1963), 60. Niebuhr's question, fundamental to his view of Christian moral responsibility, not only preceded Gustafson's and May's temporally but also was an important influence on the way in which each of these theological ethicists continued Niebuhr's work.

25. MacLeish, *J.B.*, 132.

26. Elaine Scarry, *The Body in Pain: The Making and Unmaking of the World* (Oxford: Oxford University Press, 1985).

27. Similarly, Dorothy L. Sayers, in *Mind of the Maker* (San Francisco: Harper & Row, 1979), 106–7, postulated that one can redeem evil by transmuting it into good through the medium of a creative act.

6. Finitude, Freedom, and Suffering

1. P. C. Phan, "The Lesser Evil of Theodicy," *CTSA Proceedings* 50 (1995): 192–200.

2. I do not use the term "ontic evil," although I develop the notion of finitude in a way that expands it beyond Janssens's use of "ontic evil." See Louis Janssens, "Ontic Evil and Moral Evil," in *Moral Norms and Catholic Tradition*, in *Readings in Moral Theology*, ed. Charles E. Curran and Richard A. McCormick (New York: Paulist Press, 1979), 40–93.

3. Terrence W. Tilley, *The Evils of Theodicy* (Washington, D.C.: Georgetown University Press, 1991), 219, 248.

4. Stanley Hauerwas, *Naming the Silences: God, Medicine, and the Problem of Suffering* (Grand Rapids, Mich.: Eerdmans, 1990).

5. For an excellent example of how the complexities of theodicy can be rendered in a pastorally useful manner, see Jack Wintz, "Why Must I Suffer?" *Catholic Update* (February 1987).

6. John Hick presents an excellent discussion of the Augustinian position on evil in *Evil and the God of Love* (London: Macmillan, 1966), 43–95. Augustine takes up the question in several of his writings; the most extensive consideration is in "Concerning the Nature of Good," available in *Basic Writings of St. Augustine*, 2d ed., ed. W. J. Oates (New York: Random House, 1948), 429–57. In his most explicit and medically relevant passage on this topic, Augustine argues:

> For what is that which we call evil but the absence of good? In the bodies of animals, disease and wounds mean nothing but the absence of health; for when a cure is effected, that does not mean that the evils which were present—namely the diseases and the wounds—go away from the body and exist elsewhere; they altogether cease to exist; for the wound is not a substance, but a defect in the fleshly substance—the flesh being itself a substance, and therefore something good, of which those evils—that is, privations of that good which we call health—are accidents. . . . All things that exist, therefore, seeing that the Creator of them all is supremely good, are themselves good. But, because they are not like their Creator, supremely and unchangeably good, their good may be diminished or increased. (*Enchiridion* 11–2, in W. J. Oates, ed., *Basic Writings*, 662–63)

7. *Summa Theologiae*, Blackfriars edition, ed. T. Gilly (New York: McGraw-Hill, 1966), I-I, q.2, a.3; qq. 48–49.

8. Gottfried Wilhelm Leibniz, *Theodicy: Essays on the Goodness of God, the Freedom of Man, and the Origin of Evil*, trans. E. M. Huggard (New Haven, Conn.: Yale University Press, 1952).

9. A related theory, also traceable to Augustine, is sometimes known as the "aesthetic" theory: Just as paintings require a bit of shadow to bring out the intensity of color, so the universe needs a bit of evil as contrast to show off its goodness. For a contemporary version of this, see the appendix on evil ("On Seeing") in Pierre Teilhard de Chardin, *The Phenomenon of Man* (New York: Harper & Row, 1959), 311–13. Its main thesis is that, from the viewpoint of the evolution of the species, what appears to be evil really is

not. A certain number of mistakes are required in order for the evolutionary work of art to progress properly.

10. *Five books of St. Irenaeus Against Heresies*, trans. J. Keble (London: A. D. Innes, [n.d.]). See especially 4.37–39, 5.28.3–29.1, and 5.32.1.

11. Hick, *Evil and the God of Love*; Paul Tournier, *Creative Suffering* (San Francisco: Harper & Row, 1982).

12. This criticism may represent an important point of difference between my own modified realist views and those of many theologians who have fully embraced the "turn toward the subject."

13. Barry L. Whitney, *What Are They Saying about God and Evil?* (Mahwah, N.J.: Paulist Press, 1989).

14. Hauerwas, *Naming the Silences*; Daniel Liderbach, *Why Do We Suffer?* (Mahwah, N.J.: Paulist Press, 1995); Karl Rahner, *Theological Investigations, XIX* (New York: Crossroad, 1983), 194–208; David Tracy, "Evil, Suffering, and Hope," *CTSA Proceedings* 50 (1995): 15–36.

15. Albert Camus, *The Plague*, trans. S. Gilbert (New York: Vintage, 1991).

16. Alvin Plantinga, *God, Freedom, and Evil* (Grand Rapids, Mich.: Eerdmans, 1974).

17. In general, Roman Catholicism holds a more optimistic view of human beings after original sin. See *The Catechism of the Catholic Church* (Liguori, Mo.: Liguori Publications, 1994), nos. 705, 1949–60.

18. The basic argument is as follows: True freedom implies real choice; real choice implies real possibility. For something to be a real possibility it must be naturally necessary that it should be actualized at least once. Because true freedom with respect to good and evil implies the real possibility of both good and evil, then it must be naturally necessary that evil should be actually chosen, at least once.

19. Richard Swinburne, *The Existence of God* (Oxford: Clarendon Press, 1979), 202.

20. *Catechism of the Catholic Church*, nos. 391, 414, 1521.

21. In theological circles, this enterprise is known as theological anthropology. My essentialist account may be considered one type of philosophical anthropology.

22. This is not to say that there is no such thing as attributed human dignity—i.e., aspects of human dignity that depend on how one is valued by others or how one values oneself. Rather, it is to suggest that the essentialist can hold that human dignity has an essential, intrinsic core that depends only on being human. See Daniel P. Sulmasy, "Death and Human Dignity," *Linacre Quarterly* 61 (1994): 27–36.

23. The argument is as follows: Anything that is a truly infinite, totally unconditioned being, must be singular, because if one were to suggest that there could be something other than It, but not already It, It would not be infinite. Therefore, if God is truly an infinite, unconditioned being, everything else that exists that is not God must be finite. This argument is an elaboration on a Thomistic argument in chapter 5 of *De Ente et Essentia*. See Thomas Aquinas, *On Being and Essence*, 2d ed., trans. A. Maurer (Toronto: Pontifical Institute of Medieval Studies, 1983).

24. John Paul II, "The Christian Meaning of Human Suffering" (*Salvifici Doloris*), *Origins* 13 (1984): 610–24.

25. P. J. Van der Maas, J. J. M. van Delden, and L. Pijneborg, *Euthanasia and Other Medical Decisions Concerning the End of Life* (Amsterdam: Elsevier, 1993).

26. John Paul II, "Christian Meaning of Human Suffering."

27. Readers may recognize this as a restatement of Ockham's opinion about God's power and freedom. See Frederick Copleston, *Late Medieval and Renaissance Philosophy*, in *A History of Philosophy*, vol. 3, pt. 1 (New York: Image, 1963), 106.

28. Karl Rahner, *Hominisation: The Evolutionary Origin of Man as a Theological Problem* (New York: Herder & Herder, 1965).

29. John Paul II, "Message to Pontifical Academy of Sciences on Evolution," *Origins* 26 (1996): 414–16.

30. Hick, *Evil and the God of Love*, 358 ff.

31. Swinburne, *Existence of God*, 202–3.

32. Donald Nicholl, *Holiness* (Mahwah, N.J.: Paulist Press, 1987), 145–46.

7. The Practice of Theodicy

1. Several years ago I was a member of an undergraduate's honors committee. During the course of an entire year I was unsuccessful in making this philosophy student understand that evil was a problem because of the anguish of lived suffering. It remained for him a pristinely clean, clear logical problem, solvable by logical devices. He was very smart, but suffering, I think, from what Thomas Aquinas termed "invincible ignorance," incapable of understanding that suffering is borne by human bodies and souls and that suffering can crush and destroy those bodies and souls.

2. Terrence Tilley calls this *justification* of evil one of the central "evils of theodicy." He argues that the practice of theodicy is "part of the Enlightenment obsession with reducing the muddy and mixed to the clear and distinct. But . . . for all theodicists, the practical problems remain. Indeed, they are exacerbated by the practice of distancing oneself from the reality of evils to understand how evil does not count against belief in God. The practice of theodicy valorizes the spotless hands which write about evils without being sullied by them" (Terrence Tilley, *The Evils of Theodicy* [Washington, D.C.: Georgetown University Press, 1991], 232).

3. Richard M. Zaner, *Troubled Voices: Stories of Ethics and Illness* (Cleveland: The Pilgrim Press, 1993), 43.

4. "To wrap evils in good words is to hide their viciousness, to disguise their poison, to refuse to acknowledge the rot that eats at our humanity—in short, to engage in practices which reproduce evils" (Tilley, *The Evils of Theodicy*, 213).

5. Elaine Scarry, *The Body in Pain: The Making and Unmaking of the World* (Oxford: Oxford University Press, 1985), 30.

6. Zaner relates, with gentleness and sympathy, a somewhat chilling story of a woman who chooses a therapeutic abortion, and ends up divorcing her husband because of it, when genetic testing reveals that both the unborn child and her husband carry a gene for Huntington's chorea, a disease which appears in the forties (*Troubled Voices*, 94). It is a

terrible dilemma to be in, yet I am troubled by the assumption that a life destined to end after only 40 or so years is simply not worth living.

7. Julian of Norwich, the fourteenth-century mystic, wrote: "I saw that our nature is wholly in God, in which he makes diversities flowing out of him to perform his will which nature preserves and mercy and grace restore and fulfil" (Julian of Norwich, *Showings*, trans. Edmund Colledge, O.S.A., and James Walsh, S.J. [New York: Paulist Press], 291).

8. Leo Tolstoy, "The Death of Ivan Ilych," in *The Fabric of Existentialism: Philosophical and Literary Sources*, ed. Richard Gill and Ernest Sherman (Englewood Cliffs, N.J.: Prentice-Hall, 1973), 61.

9. Life is one of Pseudo-Dionysius's names for God. "Every animal and plant is enlivened and fostered from out of it. Further, every life whatsoever—whether you speak of intellectual, rational, sensible, nutritive or generative life—every source of life, and every being of life is enlivened from the [divine life] beyond all life. . . . It is to be celebrated in terms of all living things according to the multiple fecundity of what lives as manifold, contemplated, and celebrated by every life, without lack, over full of life, self living . . . and however else one might humanly celebrate the unspeakable life" (Pseudo-Dionysius, *Divine Names and Mystical Theology*, trans. John D. Jones [Milwaukee: Marquette University Press, 1980], 857B). The significance of this way of naming God, as cause beyond being, is that God is the power of life and beauty. Death is therefore a privation of what we are empowered for by the Good beyond Being.

10. Roberta C. Bondi, *In Ordinary Time: Healing the Wounds of the Heart* (Nashville: Abingdon Press, 1996), 90.

11. Julian has a picturesque description of this: "When God was to make man's body, he took the slime of the earth, which is matter mixed and gathered from all bodily things, and of that he made man's body. But to the making of man's soul he would accept nothing at all, but made it. . . . Therefore he wants us to know that the noblest thing which he ever made is mankind, and the fullest substance and the highest power is the blessed soul of Christ. And furthermore, he wants us to know that this beloved soul was preciously knitted to him in its making, by a knot so subtle and so mighty that it is united in God. In this uniting it is made endlessly holy" (Julian of Norwich, *Showings*, 284).

12. Both traditional and process theism understand this tragic (or, in the premodern literature, aesthetic) character of creation. Thomas Aquinas, for example, said, "if all evil were prevented, much good would be absent from the universe. A lion would cease to live, if there were no slaying of animals; and there would be no patience of martyrs if there were no tyrannical persecution" (*Summa Theologica*, Q.22 a.1). This interdependence of good and evil is central to process philosophy; see, for example, John Cobb and David Griffin's *Process Theology: an Introductory Exposition* (Philadelphia: Westminster Press, 1976), in which the writers follow Whitehead in arguing that both triviality and discord are forms of evil, but that overcoming one tends to the other (75). See also Alfred North Whitehead's "Peace," in *Adventures in Ideas* (New York: Macmillan, 1933), where this point is developed more carefully.

13. Bondi, *In Ordinary Time*, 92. In this she is close to Schleiermacher, the great nineteenth-century theologian. For him, the meaning of the crucifixion rests in its power precisely to cleave the connection in experience between suffering and guilt (Friedrich

Schleiermacher, *The Christian Faith*, trans. and ed. H. R. Mackintosh and J. S. Stewart [Philadelphia: Fortress Press, 1928], 425–75).

14. "That, beautiful beyond being, is said to be

Beauty—for

    it gives beauty from itself in a manner

    appropriate to each."

—Pseudo-Dionysius, *Divine Names*, chapter IV, 703C

15. Julian of Norwich, *Showings*, 264.

16. H. Richard Niebuhr, *The Responsible Self: An Essay In Christian Moral Philosophy* (San Francisco: Harper & Row, 1963), 126.

17. Julian of Norwich, *Showings*, 295.

18. Zaner, *Troubled Voices*, 44–46.

19. Ibid., 144.

20. Ibid., 145–46.

21. Zaner describes "the ethicist's" involvement in suffering as "the occasion for highly specific talk among just these individuals with just their lives, circumstances, concerns, feelings, aims, and proposals for acting" (Zaner, *Troubled Voices*, 147).

22. This is how Shantideva describes *bodhicitta*, that is, the enlightened mind or the mind of compassion:

This is the elixir of life, born to end death in the world.

This is the inexhaustible treasure, alleviating poverty in the world.

This is the supreme medicine, curing the sickness of the world,

a tree of shelter for weary creatures staggering along the road of existence.

(Shantideva, *The Bodhicaryvartara*, trans. Kate Crosby and Andrew Skilton [Oxford: Oxford University Press, 1985], 3.28–29)

8. Rabbi, Why Does God Make Me Suffer?

[In the following, M. = Mishnah (edited c. 200 C.E.); T. = Tosefta (also edited c. 200 C.E.); J. = Jerusalem Talmud (edited c. 400 C.E.); B. = Babylonian Talmud (edited c. 500 C.E.); M.T. = Maimonides' *Mishneh Torah* (completed 1177); and S.A. = Joseph Karo's *Shulhan Arukh* (completed 1565).]

1. See, for example, Deuteronomy 10:14, Psalm 24:1. See also Genesis 14:19, 22 (where the Hebrew word for "Creator" [*koneh*] also means "Possessor," and where "heaven and earth" is a merism for those and everything in between); Exodus 20:11; Leviticus 25:23, 42, 55; Deuteronomy 4:35, 39; 32:6.

2. See, for example, Maimonides' codified rules requiring proper care of the body: M.T. *Laws of Ethics (De'ot)*, chapters 3–5.

3. B. *Shabbat* 32a; B. *Bava Kamma* 15b, 80a, 91b; M.T. *Laws of Murder* 11:4–5; S.A. *Yoreh De'ah* 116:5 gloss; S.A. *Hoshen Mishpat* 427:8–10.

4. Genesis 9:5; M. *Semahot* 2:2; B. *Bava Kamma* 91b; *Genesis Rabbah* 34:19 states that the ban against suicide includes not only cases where blood was shed, but also self-

inflicted death through strangulation and the like; M.T. *Laws of Murder* 2:3; M.T. *Laws of Injury and Damage* 5:1; S.A. *Yoreh De'ah* 345:1–3. Cf. J. David Bleich, *Judaism and Healing* (New York: KTAV, 1981), ch. 26.

5. Maimonides, in his typical clarity, states this principle explicitly when he says that "He who regulates his life in accordance with the laws of medicine with the sole motive of maintaining a sound and vigorous physique and begetting children to do his work and labor for his benefit is not following the right course. A man should aim to maintain physical health and vigor in order that his soul may be upright, in a condition to know God." M.T. *Laws of Ethics (De'ot)* 3:3.

6. The law of the Nazarite appears in Numbers 6:11; the Rabbinic derivation from that law that abstinence is prohibited appears first in B. *Ta'anit* 11a. See also M.T. *Laws of Ethics (De'ot)* 3:1.

7. *Sifra* on Leviticus 19:16; B. *Sanhedrin* 73a; M.T. *Laws of Murder* 1:14; S.A. *Hoshen Mishpat* 426.

8. For more on Judaism's general attitude toward medicine, see Elliot N. Dorff, *Matters of Life and Death: A Jewish Perspective on Modern Medical Ethics* (Philadelphia: Jewish Publication Society, 1998), ch. 2.

9. Cf. Leviticus 23:32; M. *Yoma*, ch. 8, and later rabbinic commentaries and codes based on that.

10. M. *Avot* 2:16; B. *Berakhot* 4a; B. *Eruvin* 19a; B. *Ta'anit* 11a; B. *Kiddushin* 39b; *Genesis Rabbah* 33:1; *Yalkut Ecclesiastes* 978. Among later Jewish philosophers, Saadia is the first to affirm this doctrine (*Book of Opinions and Beliefs*, Books 4 and 5), while Maimonides rejects it (*Guide for the Perplexed*, ed. Shlomo Pines [Chicago: University of Chicago Press, 1963], Part III, chapters 16–23).

11. B. *Berakhot* 5b. I would like to thank Rabbi Baruch Frydman-Kohl for suggesting the use of this source here.

12. God's promise to prevent illness if we obey His commandments: Deuteronomy 7:12–15. God serves as our Healer and, conversely, uses illness as a punishment for sin: see note 8 above.

13. B. *Shabbat* 55a; see also B. *Nedarim* 41a and B. *Sanhedrin* 101a. A tenth-century commentary put this view graphically: "If a subject sins against his ruler, a blacksmith is commanded to fashion chains in which the ruler imprisons the sinner. When a man sins against the Lord, his limbs become his fetters" (*Midrash Tadshe* 16). See also B. *Ta'anit* 11a; B. *Kiddushin* 40b; and B. *Berakhot* 5b, where some rabbis maintain that the punishment God inflicts is a product of His love, for it deters the sinner from sinning that way again.

14. B. *Bava Mezia* 58b. For examples of their medical research, see Fred Rosner, *Medicine in the Bible and Talmud* (New York: Ktav and Yeshiva, 1977).

15. B. *Berakhot* 33b.

16. See, for example, *Genesis Rabbah* 8:4 and 5, where God creates human beings despite the angels' warning that people will make bad choices.

17. Thus Maimonides, for example, says that most of our troubles come from what we inflict on ourselves, and the next largest segment comes from what other people do to us (*Guide for the Perplexed*, Part III, ch. 12, 443–45).

18. This, of course, is the theme of Job's "friends," although God in the whirlwind

(Job, ch. 38–42) denies this. It is also behind the High Holy Day liturgy's request of God to forgive our sins, "whether we know them or not."

19. This seems unconscionable to contemporary Americans. How is it just to punish children for the sins of parents? Moreover, how can God do this (cf. Exodus 34:6–7; Numbers 14:18–19) while specifically commanding people not to do so (Deuteronomy 24:16)? In part, the Bible sees this as an act of mercy on the part of God toward the parents, just as postponing payment on a credit card is understood and felt as a favor. This, of course, leaves unresolved the injustice suffered by the children. Because of this, some sources claim that God only "visits the iniquity of the parents on the children" when the children themselves continue to do the sin. Still others suggest that the unfairness is simply a fact of life, whether or not we understand it. Children, after all, prosper unjustly from the abilities and accomplishments of their parents just as much as they suffer from their parents' deficiencies, but we only complain about the latter. Cf. Jacob Milgrom, "Vertical Retribution," *Conservative Judaism* 34 (1981): 11–16; Robert Gordis, *A Faith for Moderns* (New York: Bloch, 1960), 181–82; and Elliot N. Dorff and Arthur Rosett, *A Living Tree* (Albany: State University of New York Press, 1988), 110–23.

20. A good summary of the rabbinic material on all of the above approaches can be found in A. Cohen, *Everyman's Talmud* (New York: E. P. Dutton, 1949), 110–20, 364–89.

21. Maimonides, *Guide for the Perplexed*, Part III, ch. 10–12, 438–48.

22. Mordecai M. Kaplan, *The Meaning of God in Modern Jewish Religion* (New York: Behrman House, 1937; Reconstructionist Press, 1947), 76. The rabbinic source he cites is *Genesis Rabbah* 3:6; cf. 53:4. Milton Steinberg presents this position more convincingly in his *A Believing Jew* (New York: Harcourt, Brace and Co., 1951), 13–31.

23. Harold Kushner, *When Bad Things Happen to Good People* (New York: Shocken, 1981).

24. Kaplan, *Meaning of God*, 76.

25. Ibid., 84.

26. This seems to be the message of God out of the whirlwind in chapters 38–42 of the Book of Job, and it is clearly stated in *Avot* (*Ethics of the Fathers*) 4:19; B. *Menahot* 29b; and as R. Meir's position in B. *Berakhot* 7a. Cf. Cohen, *Everyman's Talmud*, 110–20.

27. On the Holocaust: Richard L. Rubenstein, *After Auschwitz: Radical Theology and Contemporary Judaism* (Indianapolis: Bobbs-Merrill, 1966). On the nuclear threat: Richard L. Rubenstein, "Jewish Theology and the Current World Situation," *Conservative Judaism* 28 (1974): 3–25; cf. also the responses of Arthur Green and Elliot Dorff on pages 26–36 there. Rubenstein later spelled out the implications of overpopulation, world poverty, and the nuclear threat more fully in his *The Age of Triage* (Boston: Beacon Press, 1983), esp. chapters 1, 9, and 10.

28. Elliot N. Dorff, *Knowing God: Jewish Journeys to the Unknowable* (Northvale, N.J.: Jason Aronson, 1992), ch. 5.

29. *Mekhilta* on Exodus 20:23 (ed. Lauterbach, vol. 2, 277). For other instances where the biblical and rabbinic traditions attribute evil to God, see Isaiah 45:7; Lamentations 3:37–38; the instances where Satan is clearly under the control of God, such as 1 Kings 11:14, Psalms 109:6, Job 1:6; J. *Ta'anit* 65b, B. *Kiddushin* 81a–b, *Esther Rabbah* 7:13 (on Esther 3:9).

30. M. *Berakhot* 9:5 (= B. *Berakhot* 54a); cf. *Sifre Deuteronomy* 32. The Mishnah de-

rives this lesson from the phrase, "with all your might." The Malbim suggest another justification for this Mishnaic principle. Commenting on Deuteronomy 6:4–5, he notes that the *juxtaposition* of God's unity in verse 4 with the love of God in verse 5 suggests that, when we recognize God as One, we are challenged to love the Eternal as the source of all that happens to us, both good and evil.

31. *Sifre Deuteronomy,* "*Ha'azinu,*" par. 329. Since the rabbis were engaged in an unceasing war against Zoroastrian dualism, they were keenly aware, as they demonstrate in this passage, of the dangers of attributing evil to anyone or anything but the one God.

32. Despite the existence of books like Job, the Bible does not ultimately reconcile God's goodness, which it affirms often (e.g., Deuteronomy 32:4; Jeremiah 9:23; Amos 5:24; Zephaniah 3:5; Psalms 11:7, 97:2, 99:4), with the evil that God inscrutably causes or does not prevent. The Rabbis, however, attempted to construct a coherent view of these phenomena. For them, "*tov*" (good) is God's main attribute (J. *Haggigah* 77c, *Ecclesiastes Rabbah* 7:8, and *Ruth Rabbah* 3:16), and God's mercy will assert itself if a person repents (e.g., *Pesikta* 164a). God requites people according to their own measure ("*middah ke-neged middah,*" T. *Sotah* 3; J. *Sotah* 17a, b; B. *Sanhedrin* 90a, b), but the measure of good always exceeds that of evil and punishment ("*middat tovah merubbah mi-middat puraniyyut,*" *Mekhilta,* Beshalah, ed. Lauterbach, vol. 2, 113; ed. Horowitz-Robin, 166). One opinion in the tradition (B. *Berakhot* 34b), however, makes Messianic times different from our own era only in that the *political* frustration of the Jewish people would be alleviated; otherwise, we would all remain much as we are.

33. B. *Menahot* 43b. Blessings actually acknowledge God's power as well as God's goodness. Cf. B. *Berakhot* 35a: "Whoever enjoys this world's pleasures without reciting a blessing is tantamount to one who steals from God." M.T. *Laws of Blessings* 1:3–4: "The Sages instituted many blessings of praise, thanksgiving, and petition so that we will remember the Creator always . . . and respect [fear] Him"; cf. 10:26.

34. Maimonides (*Guide for the Perplexed,* Part III, ch. 12, 444) states this point even more starkly than I have:

> [Because humanity is endowed with matter], this species of evil [that comes from matter's property of coming to be and passing away] must necessarily exist. Nevertheless, you will find that the evils of this kind that befall men are very few and occur very seldom. For you will find cities, existing for thousands of years, that have never been flooded or burned. Also thousands of people are born in perfect health whereas the birth of an infirm human being is an anomaly, or at least—if someone objects to the word "anomaly" and does not use it—such an individual is very rare; for they do not form a hundredth or even a thousandth part of those born in good health.

35. Cf. Anson Laytner, *Arguing with God: A Jewish Tradition* (Northvale, N.J.: Jason Aronson, 1990).

36. For Kant, of course, it makes sense only if it is not rewarded!

37. M. *Avot* 4:2. This puts me in direct opposition to the comment in the Tosefta by Rabbi Reuben, about whom the following is told:

It happened once that Rabbi Reuben was in Tiberias on the Sabbath, and a philosopher asked him: "Who is the most hateful man in the world?" He replied, "The man who denies the Creator." "How so?" said the philosopher. Rabbi Reuben answered: "'Honor your father and mother, you shall not murder, you shall not commit adultery, you shall not steal, you shall not bear false witness against your neighbor, you shall not covet.' No man denies the derivative (i.e., the separate commandments) until he has previously denied the Root (i.e., God), and no man sins unless he has denied Him who commanded him not to commit that sin." (T. *Shevu'ot* 3:6)

I agree that it is *easier* to be motivated to observe the commandments if you think that God will punish you for not observing them and reward you if you do. As the rabbis recognized elsewhere, however, (a) that is *not* the proper motivation (M. *Avot* 1:3); (b) it does not even work out that way, at least as far as we know (cf. note 26 above), and it must, therefore, eventually lose force as a motivation; and (c) moreover, it *is* possible to observe Jewish law without a theological whipping stick—indeed, without God at all (cf. *Pesikta*, XV, ed. Buber, 120a–121b; ed. Mandelbaum, 254).

In my book, *Mitzvah Means Commandment* (New York: United Synagogue of America, 1989), I discuss at some length the multiplicity of motivations to observe the law that the Bible and rabbis delineated. They did not restrict the motivations to observe the law to divine reward and punishment, although that certainly was included.

38. Sometimes this is because people have different thresholds of pain, so it is difficult to know how much to prescribe. Other factors in this phenomenon, though, are the "John Wayne" attitude in the United States that people should "grin and bear it," and the war mentality in American medicine that overcoming disease is a battle; when it cannot be won, physicians often withdraw from the scene. This approach is part of the reason that patients request help in committing suicide. As an editorial in the *Annals of Internal Medicine* maintained, far too many people are finding that physicians "are so preoccupied with the preservation of life that they can no longer see the broader human context of their work" (cited by Terrence Monmaney, in "How We Die May Be Behind Assisted Suicide Debate," *Los Angeles Times*, January 8, 1997, A1, A9).

39. M. *Bava Kamma* 8:1, 6, 7; B. *Bava Kamma*, ch. 8 generally, esp. 84a–b, 86a–b.

40. *Zohar*, I, 229b.

41. B. *Shabbat* 127a; B. *Sotah* 14a; B. *Nedarim* 39–40b; B. *Bava Kamma* 100a; M.T. *Laws of Mourning* 14:4.

42. Rabbi Nissim Gerondi (c. 1360) is the first to mention such societies, perhaps because in earlier times Jews lived in communities sufficiently small to insure that everyone would be visited even without such a formal structure to make sure it happened. See *Encyclopedia Judaica* 14:1498.

43. B. *Nedarim* 39b–40a.

44. B. *Berakhot* 6a; 7b–8a; J. *Berakhot* 5:1; cf. M.T. *Laws of Prayer* 8:1.

45. B. *Nedarim* 41a.

46. B. *Ta'anit* 8a; cf. M.T. *Laws of Prayer* 8:1.

47. B. *Nedarim* 39b–40a.

48. M.T. *Laws of Mourning*, ch. 14; S.A. *Yoreh De'ah* 335. Other sources in English on Jewish practices regarding visiting the sick include Isaac Klein, *A Guide to Jewish Religious Practice* (New York: Jewish Theological Seminary of America, 1979), 271–72; Pesach Krauss, *Why Me? Coping with Grief, Loss, and Change* (Toronto and New York: Bantam, 1988), esp. chapters 16 and 17, 123–39; Tsvi G. Schur, *Illness and Crisis: Coping the Jewish Way* (New York: National Conference of Synagogue Youth/Union of Orthodox Jewish Congregations of America, 1987), esp. ch. 6, 66–9; Abraham S. Abraham, *Medical Halachah for Everyone* (New York: Feldheim, 1980), ch. 35, 135–38; and a pamphlet, *Bikkur Holim* (New York: Women's League for Conservative Judaism, 1992), for all the sisterhoods of Conservative congregations.

49. M.T. *Laws of Mourning* 14:6; Tosafot on B. *Shabbat* 127a; S.A. *Yoreh De'ah* 335:3, gloss.

9. To Change and to Accept in a Technological Society

1. According to *Bartlett's Familiar Quotations* (15th ed., ed. E. M. Beck [Boston: Little, Brown, 1980], 823), this prayer was written in 1943 by Reinhold Niebuhr for a service in the Congregational Church in Heath, Massachusetts. It was later printed in the newsletter of the Federal Council of Churches and, in modified form, has become the "Serenity Prayer" familiar to participants in Alcoholics Anonymous and related "twelve-step" recovery programs.

2. Albert Borgmann, *Crossing the Postmodern Divide* (Chicago: University of Chicago Press, 1992); Daniel Callahan, *Setting Limits: Medical Goals in an Aging Society* (New York: Simon & Schuster, 1987); Reed Kariam, "Technology and Its Discontents," *Civilization*, May/June 1995, 47–51; Charles Taylor, *The Ethics of Authenticity* (Cambridge: Harvard University Press, 1991).

3. The social significance I attribute to technology is not defended here. Others have already made that case, among them Albert Borgmann, *Technology and the Character of Contemporary Life* (Chicago: University of Chicago Press, 1984); Hans Jonas, *The Imperative of Responsibility: In Search of an Ethics for the Technological Age*, trans. Hans Jonas with David Herr (Chicago: University of Chicago Press, 1984); Arthur M. Melzer, "The Problem with the 'Problem of Technology,'" in *Technology in the Western Political Tradition*, ed. Arthur M. Melzer, Jerry Weinberger, and M. Richard Zinman (Ithaca, N.Y.: Cornell University Press, 1993), 287–321.

4. Emmanuel Levinas, "Useless Suffering," in *The Provocations of Levinas: Rethinking the Other*, ed. Robert Bernasconi and David Wood (London: Routledge, 1988), 156–67.

5. I shall examine Christian versions of theodicy, although attention should also be paid to Judaism and Islam in their treatment of these issues. See Ronald M. Green, "Theodicy," in *Encyclopedia of Religion*, ed. Mircea Eliade (New York: Macmillan, 1987).

6. See H. Richard Niebuhr, *The Responsible Self: An Essay in Christian Moral Philosophy* (New York: Harper & Row, 1963).

7. Peter Berger, *The Sacred Canopy: Elements of a Sociological Theory of Religion* (Garden City, N.Y.: Anchor Books, 1969); Eric Cassell, *The Nature of Suffering and the Goals of*

Medicine (New York: Oxford University Press, 1991); Clifford Geertz, *The Interpretation of Cultures: Selected Essays* (New York: Basic Books, 1973); William F. May, *The Patient's Ordeal* (Bloomington: Indiana University Press, 1991); David B. Morris, *The Culture of Pain* (Berkeley: University of California Press, 1991); Daniel Day Williams, "Suffering and Being in Empirical Theology," in *The Future of Empirical Theology*, ed. Bernard E. Meland (Chicago: University of Chicago Press, 1969), 175–94.

8. May, *Patient's Ordeal*, 2–14.

9. Niebuhr, *Responsible Self*, 55–68.

10. Cassell, *Nature of Suffering*, 30–65; Levinas, "Useless Suffering," 156–59; Williams, "Suffering and Being," 180–81.

11. Nicholas Wolterstorff, *Lament for a Son* (Grand Rapids, Mich.: Eerdmans, 1987), 69.

12. Eric Cassell, "Pain and Suffering" in *Encyclopedia of Bioethics*, rev. ed., ed. Warren Thomas Reich (New York: Simon & Schuster Macmillan, 1995), 1897–1905; Dorothee Soelle, *Suffering* (Philadelphia: Fortress Press, 1975), 61–86.

13. Berger, *Sacred Canopy*, 3–51.

14. Ibid., 55.

15. Ibid., 79.

16. Niebuhr, *Responsible Self*, 61–62.

17. Paul Ricoeur, "Evil, a Challenge to Philosophy and Theology," *Journal of the American Academy of Religion* 53 (1985): 645.

18. Langdon Gilkey, "The Christian Understanding of Suffering," *Buddhist-Christian Studies* 5 (1985): 49–65.

19. St. Augustine, *The Confessions*, 7.5, trans. F. J. Sheed (London: Sheed & Ward, 1944).

20. John Hick, *Evil and the God of Love*, rev. ed. (New York: Harper & Row, 1978).

21. Ibid., 350.

22. John Paul II, *On the Christian Meaning of Suffering* (Washington, D.C.: Office of Publishing Services, United States Catholic Conference, 1984), 32.

23. Berger, *Sacred Canopy*, 53–80; Geertz, *Interpretation of Cultures*, 87–125.

24. Soelle, *Suffering*, 19.

25. Harold Kushner, *When Bad Things Happen to Good People* (New York: Schocken Books, 1981), 136.

26. Soelle, *Suffering*, 70.

27. Melzer, "Problem with the 'Problem of Technology,'" 305, 290.

28. Alexander Barzel, "The Co-Relational Community and Technological Culture," in *Technology and Contemporary Culture*, ed. Paul T. Durbin (Dordrecht: D. Reidel, 1988), 45–62.

29. N. Bruce Hannay and Robert E. McGinn, "The Anatomy of Modern Technology: Prolegomenon to an Improved Public Policy for the Social Management of Technology," *Daedalus* 109 (1980): 25–53.

30. Hans Jonas, "Toward a Philosophy of Technology," *Hastings Center Report* 9, no. 1 (1979): 34–43.

31. Borgmann, *Technology*, 40–48.

32. Leon Kass, "Introduction: The Problem of Technology," in *Technology in the Western Political Tradition*, ed. Arthur M. Melzer, Jerry Weinberger, and M. Richard Zinman (Ithaca, N.Y.: Cornell University Press, 1993), 4–5.

33. Levinas, "Useless Suffering," 158–59.

34. Arthur Frank, *The Wounded Storyteller: Body, Illness, and Ethics* (Chicago: University of Chicago Press, 1995); Stanley Hauerwas, *Naming the Silences: God, Medicine, and the Problem of Suffering* (Grand Rapids, Mich.: Eerdmans, 1990); Morris, *Culture of Pain*.

35. Wendy Farley, *Tragic Vision and Divine Compassion: A Contemporary Theodicy* (Louisville: Westminster/John Knox Press, 1990); Kenneth Seeskin, "The Reality of Radical Evil," *Judaism* 29 (1980): 440–53; Soelle, *Suffering*; Kenneth Surin, *Theology and the Problem of Evil* (New York: Basil Blackwell, 1986).

36. Levinas, "Useless Suffering," 161–64.

37. Surin, *Theology and the Problem of Evil*, 52; see also Douglas John Hall, *God and Human Suffering: An Exercise in the Theology of the Cross* (Minneapolis: Augsburg, 1986); Soelle, *Suffering*.

38. Burton Z. Cooper, *Why, God?* (Atlanta: John Knox Press, 1988); Farley, *Tragic Vision*; Hall, *God and Human Suffering*; Hauerwas, *Naming the Silences*; Soelle, *Suffering*; Surin, *Theology and the Problem of Evil*.

39. Ricoeur, "Evil, a Challenge to Philosophy and Theology," 645.

40. Albert Camus, *The Plague* (New York: Modern Library, 1947), 117–18.

41. Melzer, "Problem with the 'Problem of Technology,'" 308–9.

42. Kass, "Introduction," 12–14.

43. Jacques Ellul, *The Technological Society*, trans. John Wilkinson (New York: Vintage Books, 1964).

44. Edward Tenner, *Why Things Bite Back: Technology and the Revenge of Unintended Consequences* (New York: Knopf, 1996), 5, 10.

45. Taylor, *Ethics of Authenticity*; Langdon Winner, "Citizen Virtues in a Technological Order," in *Technology and the Politics of Knowledge*, ed. Andrew Feenberg and Alastair Hannay (Bloomington: Indiana University Press, 1995).

46. Tenner, *Why Things Bite Back*, 254.

47. Ibid., 277.

48. Kass, "Introduction," 18.

49. Hans Jonas, "The Blessing and Burdens of Mortality," *Hastings Center Report* 22, no. 1 (1992): 34–40; Daniel Callahan, *The Troubled Dream of Life: Living with Mortality* (New York: Simon & Schuster, 1993).

50. Borgmann, *Crossing the Postmodern Divide*; Frank, *Wounded Storyteller*.

10. The Secular Problem of Evil and the Vocation of Medicine

1. John Kekes, *Facing Evil* (Princeton: Princeton University Press, 1990).

2. Peter Kivy, "Melville's *Billy* and the Secular Problem of Evil: The Worm in the Bud," *Monist* 63 (1980): 480–93.

3. Richard Powers, *Galatea 2.2* (New York: HarperCollins, 1995).

4. Ibid., 313.

5. Ibid.

6. Ibid., 314.

7. Toni Morrison, *The Bluest Eye* (New York: Holt, Rinehart & Winston, 1970).

8. A very poignant feature of *The Bluest Eye* is that Pecola cannot escape evil even in the world she creates for herself. She cannot free herself from racist-installed desires even there. Instead, she gratifies them.

9. It might be wondered whether Helen and even Pecola should count as agents in the first place. Helen, after all, is a machine and Pecola a child situated in a place that seems hostile to taking her with any kind of seriousness because of her sex, age, race, and appearance. My quick answer here is that moral agency takes many forms and is conditioned by many features of the social practices in which one is enmeshed. Helen and Pecola occupy agents' space in their social world. They just are not paradigmatic of agency and, for that reason, are not bad examples. But if this is not convincing, the remainder of the argument should not be greatly affected.

10. For a discussion of pertinent points, see Peter Unger, *Living High and Letting Die* (New York: Oxford University Press, 1996).

11. Bernard Williams, "Persons, Character and Morality," in *Moral Luck* (Cambridge: Cambridge University Press, 1981).

12. Susan Wolf, "Moral Saints," *Journal of Philosophy* 79 (1982): 419–38.

13. Shelly Kagan, *The Limits of Morality* (Oxford: Oxford University Press, 1993).

14. For a fascinating discussion of how very general obligations may be implied by a philosophical understanding of our response to drowning-child cases, see Robert Goodin, *Protecting the Vulnerable* (Chicago: University of Chicago Press, 1985). For an equally interesting discussion skeptical of philosophical generalizations drawn from such "easy rescue" cases, see Margaret Urban Walker, *Moral Understandings: A Feminist Study in Ethics* (New York: Routledge, 1997).

15. H. Tristram Engelhardt Jr., *Foundations of Bioethics*, 2d ed. (Oxford: Oxford University Press, 1996).

16. James Lindemann Nelson, "'Everything Includes Itself in Power': Power and Coherence in Engelhardt's *Foundations of Bioethics*," in *Reading Engelhardt: Essays on the Thought of H. Tristram Engelhardt, Jr.*, ed. Brendan P. Minogue, Gabriel Palmer-Fernández, and James E. Regan (Dordrecht: Kluwer Academic Press, 1997).

17. I use "mothering" in the sense pioneered by Sara Ruddick in which it does not essentially include birth-giving and thus is in principle open to women and to men. See Sara Ruddick, *Maternal Thinking* (New York: Beacon, 1989).

18. I am grateful to Hilde Lindemann Nelson for her thoughtful comments on various instantiations of this chapter.

11. God, Suffering, and Genetic Decisions

1. Jürgen Moltmann, *The Trinity and the Kingdom: The Doctrine of God*, trans. Margaret Kohl (New York: Harper & Row, 1981), 49.

2. Hastings Center, "The Goals of Medicine: Setting New Priorities," *Hastings Center Report* 26, no. 6 (1996): Siii (italics in original).

3. Ibid., S12.

4. "National Society of Genetic Counselors Code of Ethics," *Journal of Genetic Counseling* 1 (1992): 42.

5. Committee on Assessing Genetic Risks, Institute of Medicine, National Academy of Science, *Assessing Genetic Risks: Implications for Health and Social Policy*, ed. Lori B. Andrews, Jane E. Fullarton, Neil A. Holtzman, and Arno G. Motulsky (Washington, D.C.: National Academy Press, 1994), 16.

6. "Principles," in *Genetic Counseling Principles in Action: A Casebook*, ed. Joan H. Marks, Audrey Heimler, Elsa Reich, Nancy S. Wexler, and Susan E. Ince (White Plains, N.Y.: March of Dimes Birth Defects Foundation, 1989), 138, 140.

7. Roger Lincoln Shinn, *The New Genetics: Challenges for Science, Faith, and Politics* (Wakefield, R.I.: Moyer Bell, 1996), 51.

8. Arthur Peacocke, *Theology for a Scientific Age: Being and Becoming—Natural, Divine and Human* (Minneapolis: Fortress Press, 1993), 126.

9. John C. Polkinghorne, *One World* (Princeton, N.J.: Princeton University Press, 1986), 67.

10. Paul Fiddes, *The Creative Suffering of God* (Oxford: Clarendon Press, 1988), 16.

11. Ibid., 17.

12. Jürgen Moltmann, *The Crucified God: The Cross of Christ as the Foundation and Criticism of Christian Theology*, trans. R. A. Wilson and John Bowden (New York: Harper & Row, 1974), 227.

13. Ibid., 152.

14. Ibid., 246.

15. See Lisa Sowle Cahill, "The Embryo and the Fetus: New Moral Contexts," *Theological Studies* 54 (1993): 124–42; and Congregation for the Doctrine of the Faith, "Instruction on Respect for Human Life in Its Origin and on the Dignity of Procreation," *Origins* 16 (1987): 702.

16. Augustine, *City of God*, trans. Henry Bettenson (London: Penguin Books, 1972), 1055 (book 22.14).

17. Gregory of Nyssa, "On Infants' Early Deaths," trans. William Moore and Henry Austin Wilson, in *Select Writings and Letters of Gregory, Bishop of Nyssa*, A Select Library of Nicene and Post-Nicene Fathers of the Christian Church, Second Series, ed. Philip Schaff and Henry Wace, vol. 5 (Grand Rapids, Mich.: Eerdmans, 1979), 373–74.

18. Austin Farrer, *Love Almighty and Ills Unlimited* (Garden City, N.Y.: Doubleday, 1961), 166.

19. United Methodist Church, "Genetic Science," *The Book of Resolutions of the United Methodist Church 1992* (Nashville: United Methodist Publishing House, 1992), 325–38; United Church of Christ, "Pronouncement on the Church and Genetic Engineering," *Social Policy Actions*, General Synod 17, June 29–July 4, 1989 (Cleveland: Office for Church and Society, 1989), 29–31; World Council of Churches, *Biotechnology: Its Challenges to the Churches and the World* (Geneva: World Council of Churches, Subunit on Church and Society, 1989).

20. Ronald Cole-Turner and Brent Waters, *Pastoral Genetics: Theology and Care at the Beginning of Life* (Cleveland: The Pilgrim Press, 1996), 131.

12. Bioethics and the Challenge of Theodicy

1. Addressing theodicy in relation to bioethics is not the same as addressing the charge of medicine itself in relation to suffering, although the two are certainly related, as I make clear below.

2. I recognize the philosophical difficulties of and anthropological challenges to attempts to identify common or universal features of any aspect of human experience. Clearly, suffering is understood differently in different cultural and religious contexts. My discussion should be understood, therefore, as pertaining to the Western context, in which suffering has been understood as a problem to which theodicies are an intelligible means of response.

3. Erich H. Loewy, *Suffering and the Beneficent Community: Beyond Libertarianism* (Albany: State University of New York Press, 1991), 8.

4. Eric J. Cassell, "Recognizing Suffering," *Hastings Center Report* 21, no. 3 (1991): 25.

5. Ibid., 26.

6. Stanley Hauerwas, *Suffering Presence: Theological Reflections on Medicine, the Mentally Handicapped, and the Church* (Notre Dame, Ind.: University of Notre Dame Press, 1986), 28.

7. Cassell, "Recognizing Suffering," 25.

8. Ibid., 26.

9. Hauerwas, *Suffering Presence*, 28.

10. Loewy, *Suffering and the Beneficent Community*, 3.

11. Alasdair MacIntyre, *Whose Justice? Which Rationality?* (Notre Dame, Ind.: University of Notre Dame Press, 1988), 362.

12. In this chapter I use the term *medicine* to capture not merely clinical care but also medical research and education.

13. Gerald P. McKenny, *To Relieve the Human Condition: Bioethics, Technology, and the Body* (Albany: State University of New York Press, 1997), 2. For a related perspective on this issue, see Leon Kass, *Toward a More Natural Science* (New York, Free Press, 1985), 157–86.

14. "The Goals of Medicine: Setting New Priorities," *Hastings Center Report* 26, no. 6 (1996): S12.

15. Hauerwas, *Suffering Presence*, 23–36.

16. Eric Cassell, "The Sorcerer's Broom," *Hastings Center Report* 23, no. 6 (1993): 32–39.

17. Aldous Huxley, *Brave New World and Brave New World Revisited* (New York: Harper & Row, 1965), 183.

18. Ibid., 184.

19. Hauerwas, *Suffering Presence*, 25.

20. McKenny, *To Relieve the Human Condition*, 10.

21. Gilbert Meilaender, *Body, Soul, and Bioethics* (Notre Dame, Ind.: University of Notre Dame Press, 1995), 52.

22. Hauerwas, *Suffering Presence*, 33–34.

23. McKenny, *To Relieve the Human Condition*, 2.

24. It might be objected that the development of resources by which to answer the problems of suffering lies squarely within the traditions that the patient or society should appeal to, rather than within bioethics. Rather than highlighting a shortcoming of bioethics, the criticism might go, my argument points precisely to its strength, namely, ensuring that persons are properly respected so that they can appeal to the particular traditions that inform their own suffering, without interference from competing traditions.

In response, I would first return to my point that bioethics is not neutral with respect to the moral traditions that might inform our questions about the meaning of suffering and about what we should allow ourselves to suffer from. It reinforces a view of persons as primarily rational agents and, as certain debates in bioethics—such as those surrounding definitions of futility and the status of embryos for research—illustrate, substantive policy conclusions are reached on that basis (see Meilaender, *Body, Soul, and Bioethics*, on this point). In addition, the influence of bioethics on policy making and on public definitions of bioethical issues provides little guidance beyond the thin resources I have already articulated.

25. See chapter 9, Per Anderson, "To Change and to Accept in a Technological Society."

26. See chapter 6, Daniel P. Sulmasy, "Finitude, Freedom, and Suffering."

27. See, for example, chapter 1, Larry D. Bouchard, "Holding Fragments."

28. Stanley Hauerwas, *Naming the Silences: God, Medicine, and the Problem of Suffering* (Grand Rapids, Mich.: Eerdmans, 1990), 53.

29. McKenny, *To Relieve the Human Condition*.

30. I develop this latter point more fully in "The Idea of Progress and the Goals of Medicine," in *The Goals of Medicine: The Forgotten Issue in Health Care Reform*, ed. Mark J. Hanson and Daniel Callahan (Washington, D.C.: Georgetown University Press, 1999).

31. McKenny, *To Relieve the Human Condition*, 217.

Conclusion: Pain Seeking Understanding

1. David Morris, *The Culture of Pain* (Berkeley: University of California Press, 1991), 254.

2. David Barnard, "Religion and Medicine: A Meditation on Lines by A. J. Heschel," *Soundings* 68 (1985): 458.

3. Richard Selzer, *Mortal Lessons: Notes on the Art of Surgery* (New York: Touchstone Books, Simon & Schuster, 1987), 47–48.